Veterinary Clinical Diagnostic Techniques

NIPA® GENX ELECTRONIC RESOURCES & SOLUTIONS P. LTD.
New Delhi-110 034

About the Authors

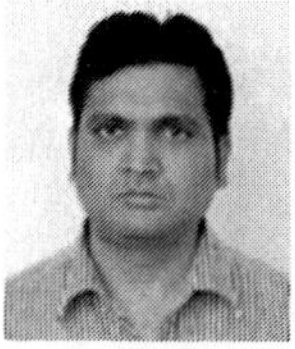

Dr. Rajesh Kumar Verma, born in the Ambedkar Nagar district of Uttar Pradesh, graduated from the DUVASU, Mathura in the year 2010 and received his master's degree and Ph.D. degree in Veterinary Microbiology from the College of Veterinary Science and Animal Husbandry, Narendra Deva University of Agriculture and Technology, Kumarganj, Faizabad. In addition to receiving the Adarsh Vidya Saraswati Rastriya Puruskar, Scientist of the Year Award, Young Scientist Award, and the Outstanding Achievement Award in Veterinary Microbiology, Dr. Verma also received a gold medal in his M.V.Sc. degree and the best thesis award in his Ph.D. degree program. He has published many books along with numerous research and clinical articles in different national and international journals. Dr. Verma is currently working as an Assistant Professor in the College of Veterinary Science and Animal Husbandry, Acharya Narendra Deva University of Agriculture and Technology, Kumarganj, Ayodhya (U.P.). He reorganised as well as re-established the clinical laboratory in the Department of Teaching Veterinary Clinical Complex as per the recommendations of the Veterinary Council of India.

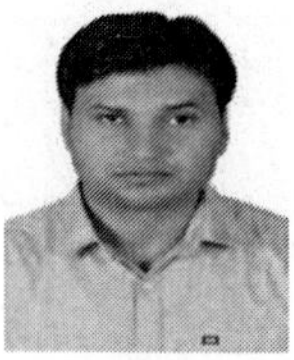

Dr. Saurabh, born in Ambedkar Nagar district of Uttar Pradesh, graduated in the year 2014, masters degree in the year 2016 and PhD in 2021 in the discipline of veterinary gynaecology and obstetrics from Acharya Narendra Deva University of agriculture and technology, kumarganj, Ayodhya. He has qualified ICAR-NET 2017 and 2018. Dr Saurabh is chancellor and vice chancellor gold medallion in M.V.Sc degree and also awarded outstanding thesis award, young scholars award, he has published different chapters in different books, many research/clinical and popular articles in different National and international journals. Presently working as assistant professor in the International Institute of veterinary education and research, Bahu Rohtak Haryana affiliated to Lala Lajpat Rai University of veterinary and animal science, Hisar.

Veterinary Clinical Diagnostic Techniques

Rajesh Kumar Verma
Assistant Professor
Department of Veterinary Clinical Complex
College of Veterinary Sciences & Animal Husbandary
Acharya Narendra Deva University of Agriculture and Technology
Kumarganj, Ayodhya
Uttar Pradesh

Saurabh
Assistant Professor
International Institute of Veterinary Education and Research
NH 10, Near Village Bahu Akbarpur
Bahu-Akbarpur, Haryana

NIPA® GENX ELECTRONIC RESOURCES & SOLUTIONS P. LTD.
New Delhi-110 034

NIPA® GENX ELECTRONIC
RESOURCES & SOLUTIONS P. LTD.

101,103, Vikas Surya Plaza, CU Block
L.S.C.Market, Pitam Pura, New Delhi-110 034
Ph : +91 11 27341616, 27341717, 27341718
E-mail: newindiapublishingagency@gmail.com
website: www.nipabooks.com

For customer assistance, please contact
Phone: + 91-11-27 34 17 17
Fax: + 91-11-27 34 16 16
E-Mail: feedbacks@nipabooks.com

ISBN: 978-93-95763-14-1

NIPA® also publishes books in a variety of electronic formats. Some content that appears in print may not be available in electronic books, and vice versa.

Composed and Designed by NIPA®.

Acknowledgements

We would like to openly express our gratitude to Dr. Sonu Jaiswal (Associate Professor, Veterinary Clinical Complex), for his insightful comments made while the manuscript was being prepared.

We would like to extend our sincere gratitude to Dr. A. K. Gangwar (Professor and Head of the Department of Surgery and Radiology), Dr. Sushant Srivastava (Professor and Head of the Department of Gynaecology and Obstetrics) and P. S. Pramanik (Dean of the College of Veterinary Science and Animal Husbandry) for their various applied and on-going encouragement to the completion of this book, which would have been possible without the continuous support of the members of our family's.

I express my indebtedness to my father Sri. R.S. Verma, this accomplishment would not have been possible without their support. He has always been a steady source of inspiration, encouragement, and a light in all the dark moments. My esteemed mother, Smt. Shobhawati Verma, deserves all the credit for my success. She offered me sound direction, a quality education, and the best advice from a young age, which is how I arrived right here. I want to express my gratitude to my wife Rachana, my son Tejas, and my daughter Aaradhya for their constant cooperation and assistance in the writing of this book.

Dr. Rajesh Kumar Verma

Finally I extend my acknowledgement with heartiest gratitude, the support and love of my family. It is like a drop in the ocean of words that can never reach its mark to acknowledge infinite love, blessings, sacrifices and constant encouragement of my uncle (Sh. Bal Govind Verma), aunty (Late Shreemati Verma), father (Dr. Jai Govind Verma) and mother (Smt. Urmila Verma) who have been the sole source of inspiration for me to proceed ahead in my life. I would like to express special thanks to my soul mate Jyoti Verma, for her close co-operation, moral support, graceful endurance and persistent endeavor which helped me successfully prepare this useful book.

Dr. Saurabh

Preface

Any animal husbandry system's production is highly sensitive to the health of the herd. For farmers and livestock in general, deviations from the maintenance of optimal herd health can have serious repercussions. Infectious diseases in animals and birds, both emerging and endemic, are a severe economic loss for our nation's distinctive sector. Disease diagnosis is a requirement for both containing and controlling such outbreaks.

We wrote this book in the expectation of providing undergraduate veterinary students who are adopting the Veterinary Council of India syllabus and veterinarians who are engaged in diagnostic laboratory services with significant and specific information. With limited resources, our field veterinarians can quickly detect illnesses using a few easy approaches. This laboratory manual has been created to provide comprehensive knowledge and information on selection of suitable samples, appropriate collection procedure, proper dispatch method, and diagnosis of microbial and parasitic agents, clinical pathology, and histopathology from a single source, helping to overcome the challenges frequently encountered in field laboratories. To improve the effectiveness of therapies and reduce the indiscriminate use of antibiotics, a veterinarian with knowledge and experience in laboratory diagnosis is needed immediately. Formats for common disease diagnosis and reporting, as well as the contact information for diagnostic firms and labs, are also provided. In order for procedures to be used by a variety of laboratory personnel, including veterinary officers, students, and technicians, procedures are briefly described in simple language for assessing the condition of an animal's health.

It is hoped that, this book on "**Veterinary Clinical Diagnostic Techniques**" would immensely benefits its users in the field of disease diagnosis.

Authors

Contents

Acknowledgements ..... *v*

Preface ..... *vii*

1. Collection, Labeling, Transportation and Preservation of Body Fluid Samples 1
   Rajesh Kumar Verma

2. Clinical Significance and Interpretation of Serum Glucose 19
   Rajesh Kumar Verma and Saurabh

3. Clinical Significance and Interpretation of Serum Protein 25
   Saurabh

4. Clinical Significance and Interpretation of Serum Lipid Profile and Serum Ketone Bodies 31
   Saurabh

5. Clinical Significance and Interpretation of Serum Minerals 35
   Rajesh Kumar Verma

6. Clinical Significance and Interpretation of Serum Electrolytes 39
   Rajesh Kumar Verma

7. Clinical Significance and Interpretation of Serum Creatinine, Urea (Bun) and Uric Acid 47
   Rajesh Kumar Verma

8. Urine Examination: Clinical Significance and Interpretation 51
   Saurabh

9. Clinical Hematology in Veterinary Practice 67
   Rajesh Kumar Verma

10. Parasitic Diseases: Laboratory Evaluation and Diagnosis of Samples 87
Rajesh Kumar Verma

11. Laboratory Diagnosis of Protozoal Infection 91
Saurabh

12. Examination of Skin Scraping 95
Saurabh

Appendix 99

1

Collection, Labeling, Transportation and Preservation of Body Fluid Samples

Rajesh Kumar Verma

Collection of Blood

Objective: To diagnose the existing disease condition, if any.

Types of blood collection

- **Arterial sampling**: In order to measure arterial blood gases, an arterial blood sample is taken from an artery. Only veterinary professionals who are legally permitted to do so for their work in their country and who have proven their expertise via formal training should take arterial blood samples.
- **Venipuncture sampling**: The most used method of taking blood from humans and animals is venipuncture. Collection occurs from a superficial vein near the surface that is not very close to any large nerves.
- **Fingerstick sampling**: A lancet is used to take one or two drops of capillary blood from a finger in "fingerstick technique," which is a minimally invasive procedure. It is also known as blood microsampling or finger-prick sampling. For laboratory analysis, 5–30 µl of blood can be drawn from a fingertip using the fingerstick technique.

The appropriate blood collection volume and procedure should be chosen after taking into account a number of parameters. These consist of:

- The species that will be sampled
- The animal's size that will be sampled
- Age and condition of the animal being sampled
- The smallest volume necessary for analysis
- The required sampling frequency
- The expertise and background of the team handling the collection
- The appropriateness of sedation or anesthesia

Requirement for blood collection

When drawing blood, the minimal equipment needed comprises

- Gloves
- Sprit and 70% ethanol to clean the area
- Tourniquet
- Collection tubes
- Tube holder
- Sterilized syringes and needles
- Cotton and gauze
- Tape

Phlebotomist should be completely knowledgeable about the variety of tubes, needles, etc.

Blood Collection steps

Phlebotomy is the process of making an incision with a needle in a vein. The procedure is known venipuncture.

- Complete the requisition form and label the tubes
- Select vein site
- Clean the area (with 70% isopropyl alcohol wipes) Inject the needle
- Perform the venipuncture

Time of collection of bold

- Early in the morning preferably 12 hrs after feeding
- Whole blood is preferred when estimation of complete blood cell count (CBC), blood ammonia, CO_2, pyruvic acid, pH and lactate is necessitated

Plasma and serum

Plasma

Starting with whole blood, coagulation is stopped and all components are retained in suspension if an anticoagulant is introduced immediately after collection. All the components will settle out when this blood sample is left alone without mixing it. Cells that are heavier will sink to the bottom. As a result, a clear liquid is obtained at the top. Plasma has all the essential elements of blood without the cells, makes up this clear upper layer. A layer of white blood cells known as the buffy coat develops between the plasma and red blood cells during centrifugation. Fibrinogen remains in the plasma.

The liquid component of the blood is called plasma. It has fibrinogen, a clotting agent that stops an excessive blood flow during an injury. Additionally, it contains proteins that aid in delivering nutrients like glucose to various regions of the body.

Plasma is taken from the upper layer of the cell during centrifugation and aids in the regulation of body temperature and blood pressure. It is separated to lengthen its shelf life to years and to enable moving it from one place to another easy.

Separation of Plasma

- Blood plasma is prepared by spinning a tube of fresh blood containing an anti-coagulant in a centrifuge until the blood cells fall to the bottom of the tube.
- Plasma is the virtually cell-free supernatant of blood containing anticoagulant obtained after centrifugation.
- Centrifuge the anticoagulated blood (citrated, EDTA or heparinized blood) for at least 15 minutes at 2000 to 3000g to obtain cell-free plasma.

Serum

Blood serum is blood plasma without fibrinogen or the other clotting factors (i.e., whole blood minus both the cells and the clotting factors).

The clotting factors encourage clot formation if we don't add any anti-coagulants. Red blood cells are effectively removed from the plasma as a solid mass by these clots, which use fibrinogen as a clotting agent. The most frequently utilized sample in research is serum, which makes up a bigger portion of blood than plasma. This results in more volume per unit of blood, at least in part because it removes the unwanted red blood cells more effectively.

Separation of serum

- Allow the blood to clot.
- Loosen the clot slowly and centrifuge the supernatant fluid for at least 10 minutes at a minimum speed of 1500g.
- By using a pipette, separate the serum from blood cells and store it in a clean and dry test tube.
- When separating serum or plasma, the temperature should not drop below 15°C or exceed 24°C.

Advantage of using plasma the fallowing aspects support the preferential use of plasma versus serum in laboratory.

1. **Time saving**: Plasma samples can be centrifuged directly after sample collection, unlike serum, in which coagulation is completed after 30 minutes.
2. **Higher yield**: 15 to 20% more in volume of plasma than of serum can be isolated from the same volume of blood.
3. **Prevention of coagulation-induced changes**: The coagulation process changes the concentrations of numerous constituents of the extra-cellular fluid beyond the maximum allowable limit. The changes are induced by the following mechanisms:
   - Increase in the concentrations of platelet components in serum as compared to plasma (e.g. potassium, phosphate, magnesium, aspartate aminotransferase, lactate dehydrogenase, serotonin, neuron specific enolase, Zinc).
   - Decrease in the concentration of constituents in serum as a result of cellular metabolism and the coagulation process (glucose, total protein, platelets).
   - Certain constituents should only be measured in plasma (e.g. neuron specific enolase, serotonin, ammonia) to obtain clinically relevant results.

Disadvantages of Plasma over serum

The addition of anticoagulants can interfere with certain analytical methods or change the concentration of the constituents to be measured:

- **Contamination with cations:** Interference in NH4+, Li+, Na+, and K+ assays caused by metals competing with EDTA and citrate (e.g. Inhibition of alkaline phosphate activity by zinc binding, inhibition of metallo-proteinases, inhibition of metal-dependent cell activation in function tests, binding of calcium (ionized) to heparin.
- **Interference by fibrinogen in heterogeneous immune assay**
- **Inhibition of metabolic catalytic reactions heparin**: e.g., Taq polymerase in the polymerase chain reaction (PCR).
- Inference in the distribution of ions between the intracellular and extracellular space (e.g. Cl^-, NH_4^+) by EDTA, citrate.
- Serum electrophoresis can be performed only after pre-treatment of induced coagulation in plasma.

Prevention of Hemolysis during blood collection

Hemolysis is the breaking of the red blood cells (RBC's) membrane, causing the release of the hemoglobin and other internal components into red tinge in surrounding fluid. Hemolysis is visually detected by showing a pink to red tinge in serum or plasma. Hemolysis is a common occurrence seen in serum samples and may compromise the laboratory's test parameters. Hemolysis can occur from two sources:

In-vivo hemolysis may be due to pathological conditions, such as autoimmune hemolytic anemia or transfusion reaction.

In-vitro hemolysis may be due to improper specimen collection, specimen processing or specimen transport.

Causes

a) Specimen Collection

i) Evacuated Tubes

- An improper choice for the vein to be punctured.
- Hemolysis could result from cleaning the venipuncture site with alcohol and not allowing it to dry.
- Slow blood flow during venipuncture can be a sign of occlusion caused by the needle's lumen being too close to the vein's inner wall, which can lead to hemolysis.
- The use of a small-bore needle can result in a significant vacuum force being applied to the blood, which can put the red blood cells under shear stress and lead to their rupture.
- Hemolysis may occur if a big bore needle is used because the blood may flow through the needle much more quickly and forcefully.

ii) Syringe Draws

- When utilizing a large bore needle, over-retracting the syringe plunger can create enough pressure for hemolysis to occur during collection. The pressure could be higher than that of a typical evacuated tube.
- Forcing blood into a tube by pressing down on the syringe plunger could result in hemolysis and create a positive pressure inside the tube that could drive the stopper off.

iii) Catheters Due to blood frothing from a loose connection of the blood collecting assemblies, hemolysis is more common when blood is obtained from a peripheral catheter.

b) Specimen Processing

- Hemolysis may result from the vigorous mixing or shaking of a specimen.
- Serum fibrin can occur hemolysis if the appropriate period of time to let the serum samples clot is not followed.
- RBCs may burst when applicator sticks are used to remove the fibrin, leading to hemolysis.
- Hemolysis may happen, if serum or plasma is exposed to cells for an extended period of time.
- RBC rupture and hemolysis can be brought on by exposure to extreme heat or cold.

c) Specimen Transport

Hemolysis might happen from mechanism trauma during transport when a pneumatic tube system is used. Variable system characteristics include length, speed, the number of times the specimen is moved, the number of angles or turns the system is employed, and other factors.

Effects of Hemolysis

Hemolysis can have an impact on test outcomes across all lab disciplines, but particularly in chemistry. Due to leakage of red cell components like lactate dehydrogenase and potassium, hemolysis may cause certain analyses to be performed more frequently or may interfere with the test procedure (e.g. spectrophotometric methods). Depending on the degree of hemolysis and the particular test method being performed, interference levels will vary. Hemolysis is a frequent reason for laboratory specimen rejection, necessitating a new specimen draw. Currently, automated evaluations of serum indices, such as the hemolysis index (HI), can be done by chemical analyzers. They offer highly repeatable quantitative measurement, standardizing the identification of hemolyzed specimens in the process.

Corrective Measures

- Use the proper needle size while drawing blood
- The choice of the needle gauge size is dependent on the patient's physical characteristics and the amount of blood to be drawn. Avoid using a needle that is too small or too large.
- Let the antiseptic at the venipuncture site dry completely.
- Without touching, allow the venipuncture site to air dry. The venipuncture site should be warmed up to promote blood flow.

- Avoid drawing the syringe plunger back too forcefully when collecting blood with a needle and syringe.
- Avoid pushing the plunger too forcefully when collecting blood.
- Ensure all blood collection assemblies are fitted securely, to avoid frothing.
- To induce coagulation, hold the tube upright at room temperature for 15-30 minutes. Then keep it at 4°C.
- To induce coagulation, hold the tube upright at room temperature for 15-30 minutes.
- Then keep it at 4°C. Within four hours of sample collection, centrifuge samples to separate the serum.
- Transfer serum to a sample tube (cryovial) and keep at 4°C if tests are run within 48 hours of collection.
- Aliquot the sample if tests will be run more than 48 hours following collection.
- If tests will be performed more than 48 hours after collection, aliquot samples and store at -20°C or lower

Commonly used anticoagulants

S.No.	Anticoagulant	Amount (per 10 ml blood)	Mode of action	Advantages
1.	Heparin	1-2 mg	Inhibition of thrombin activity	Least effect on size and haemolysis of RBCs
2.	Na-oxalate	20 mg	Chelation of Calcium	Used mainly from prothrombin time
3.	Na-citrate	10-20 mg	Chelation of Calcium	Used for blood transfusion
4.	Na-Fluoride	100mg	Prevents glycolysis by inhibiting glycolytic enzyme	Blood sugar test
5.	Ethylene diamine tetra-acetic acid (EDTA)	10-20mg	Chelation of Calcium	For routine haematology

Alterations caused on by long-term preservation of blood in EDTA

Haematological examinations

- **Packed cell volume:** increases as a result of RBC enlargement
- **Osmotic fragility:** increases in osmotic fragility
- **Platelet levels and total leucocyte count:** both gradually dropped.

Blood smear

- **RBCs:** Show crenation and spherocytic alterations in a blood smear.
- **Neutrophils:** Nuclear lobe separation, granule loss, and plasma vacuoles
- **Monocytes and lymphocytes:** Have irregular nuclear lobulation and cytoplasmic vacuoles.
- **Platelets:** Disintegration of platelets.

Blood collection sited

Animal	Site	Needle size
Cattle/ Buffalo	Jugular vein	16 gauze
Sheep	Jugular vein	18 gauze
Goat	Jugular vein	18 gauze
Camel	Jugular vein	18 gauze
Horse	Jugular vein	16 gauze
Dog	Cephalic vein, Recurrent tarsal vein, Saphenous vein	20-22 gauze,20 gauze
Cat	Cephalic vein, Jugular vein	18 gauze
Pig	Ear vein,Anterior venacava	20-22 gauze18 gauze
Poultry	Wing vein, heart	20 gauze
Mice	Retro-orbital plexus, cardiac puncture (Terminal), Tail clipping, Saphenous vein	Capillary tube24 gauzeScissors 24 gauze
Rat	Retro-orbital plexus, cardiac puncture	Capillary tube24 gauze
Guinea pig	Cardiac (anesthetized only), anterior venacava / subclavian vein	20-22 gauze
Rabbits	Cardiac (anesthetized only), marginal ear vein	18 gauze
Rhesus monkey	Cephalic vein, Saphenous vein	20-22 gauze
Hamsters	Saphenous vein cardiac puncture	22-27 gauze

Storage

- At room temp, blood can be kept up to 4 hours.
- At 4ºC, blood can be kept up to 24 hours.
- At -20ºC, blood can be kept up to 3 months.
- Whole blood should be kept in refrigerator at 4-6ºC ± 2 up to 35 days. Red cells in additive solutions can be stored up to 42 days.
- Fresh Frozen Plasma (FFP) can be stored up to one year at -30ºC or lower. Due care should be taken to maintain sterilely of blood and blood components by keeping all storage areas clean.

Short-term Storage

Routine blood storage is limited to several weeks (5 weeks for WBC, 6 weeks for RBC), and involves refrigeration but usually not freezing.

Long-term Storage

Cryopreservation of red blood cells is done to store rare units, usually for up to 3 years. Very rare units may be kept even longer. The cells are incubated in a glycerol solution which acts as a cryoprotectant (antifreeze) within the cells. The units are then placed in special sterile containers in a freezer at very cold temperatures. The exact temperature depends on the glycerol concentration.

Transport

It is necessary to maintain the cold chain at all times during transportation and storage. Proper insulted carry boxes should be used during transportation of blood. The ice in use, should be clean and should not come in direct contact with blood bags.

Types of blood tests

A. Biochemical analysis

B. Molecular profiles

   a) Protein electrophoresis

   b) Western blot

   c) Polymerase chain reaction

   d) Northern blot (RNA) diseases

   e) Sexually transmitted

C. Cellular evaluation

   a) Full blood count (or "complete blood count")

   b) Hematocrit and mean corpuscular volume (MCV)

   c) Erythrocyte sedimentation rate (ESR)

D. **Cross-matching:** Determination of blood type for blood transfusion or transplants.

E. **Blood cultures-** Blood culture are commonly taken if infection is suspected. Positive cultures and resulting sensitivity results are often useful in guiding treatment.

Collection of urine

Objective: For diagnosis of renal disease, diabetes mellitus, presence of urinary calculi, jaundice, ascites, edema, hematuria, hemoglobinuria etc.

Urine collection methods

1. Free catch collection of urine

Urine samples from free-catch are simple to obtain. A clean container with a tight-fitting lid should be used to collect urine. Animal owners should not use home-made containers that can include impurities like detergent, food, or pharmaceuticals that could change the results of a chemical reaction.

Urine samples are generally taken when an animal normally voids the urine. Samples can also be taken manually compressing the bladder and stimulating the urethra through the vulva (in cattle, buffalo, sheep, and goats). An interim sample is preferred. A voided free-catch sample has the drawback of being potentially contaminated with particles, bacteria, and cells from the vaginal tract, external skin, and distal urethra.

2. Catheterization

Although the external genital region and the distal urethral orifice are aseptically prepared and the urine bladder is catheterized, contamination of the sample is still possible. Additionally, catheterization increases the chances that red cells and transitional cells will be present in the sample because of the minor trauma it causes as it passes through the urethra, which increases the risk of iatrogenic urinary tract infections.

3. Cytocentosis

When collecting a voided, or free-catch, aliquot is not preferable, a common clinical method called cystocentesis is used to obtain a sample of urine directly from the urinary bladder of dogs and cats. When obtaining bladder urine for culture purposes, the technique is advised when evaluating the importance of cells or bacteria in the urine. In small animals, cystocentesis of the urinary bladder is typically simple to perform. In urine samples obtained through cystocentesis, a slight blood contamination may be visible. The possibility of urine leakage or haemorrhage during cystocentesis should not prevent the practitioner from performing cystocentesis in the great majority of patients, but the incidence of these problems is incredibly rare.

Preservation

Urine samples should be examined immediately after collection.

a) **Refrigeration at 4^0 C-**
   - Does not interfere with chemical tests
   - Prevents bacterial growth for 24 hours

b) Thymol @ 100 mg/100 ml of urine (it may give false reaction for albumin).

c) Formalin @1 drop/ 10 ml of urine.

Choice of preservative

a) No preservatives or refrigeration is necessary if planning to assay for heavy metals.

b) **Refrigeration** only is enough for amylase, total protein, electrolytes.

c) **Sodium carbonate** and protection from light are required for all porphyrin studies.

d) **Hydrochloric acid** is recommended for calcium, and phosphorus.

e) **Glacial acetic acid** is recommended for most steroids and catecholamine metabolites.

f) **Boric acid** is recommended for uric acid, creatinine, amino acids, and a few steroids (estradiol, cortisol). It may inhibit growth of *Pseudomonas* spp and affect a number of test strip reactions.

Container

Sterile polypropylene container.

Collection of faeces

Objective: examination of parasites, Indication of jaundice, hepatitis, anemia, presence of blood.

Methods of faecal collection

- Samples of faeces for parasitological examination should ideally be taken from the rectum. Wearing appropriate disposable gloves is recommended. Collecting from larger animals is simpler than collecting from smaller animals.
- A moistened finger can be inserted into the rectum and massaged until the external sphincter relaxes to cause defecation in smaller animals like lambs. Samples should be collected from a variety of randomly chosen or worm-affected animals, depending on the circumstances of the herd being examined.

- Faecal samples cannot be obtained directly from the cloaca during the testing of chickens. If a particular bird needs to be evaluated, it should be caged separately, cloacal swabs should be used for collection of faecal samples, or any recent droppings should be gathered. The fresh droppings can be taken from the bird if an individual bird assessment is not necessary from the poultry house.

Precautions in faecal sample collection

- Place the stool in a container that is dry, clean, and leak-proof. Ensure that the container doesn't contain any urine, water, soil, or other substances.
- Fresh faeces must to be examined, processed, or preserved immediately. When preservatives are unavailable, the only specimens eligible for testing are those kept in refrigeration; these specimens are only suitable for antigen testing.
- The specimen should be preserved as soon as possible. If utilizing a commercial collection kit, follow by the directions that came with it. If kits are not available, the specimen should be separated into two portions, each to be preserved in PVA (polyvinyl alcohol) and 10% formalin, respectively, in appropriate containers. Three volumes of the preservative should be mixed with one volume of the faeces sample.
- Make sure the preservative is thoroughly combined with the specimen. Forming stools must be thoroughly broken apart.
- Make that the containers storing the samples are well sealed. Use parafilm or other appropriate reinforcement material. The container should be covered with a plastic bag.
- The stool samples will not be suitable for testing if you use certain medications or chemicals. Before administering these medications, the specimens should be collected, or else collection must be postponed until after the effects have worn off. These include antacids, kaolin, mineral oil and other oily materials, non-absorbable antidiarrheal medications, barium or bismuth (effects take 7–10 days to clear up), antibacterial medicines (take 2–3 weeks to work), and gallbladder dyes (3 weeks).
- If the initial test is negative, specimen collection might need to be repeated. If at all feasible, it is best to analyses three specimens that were passed at 2-3 day intervals.

Preservation

When stool samples cannot be inspected within the allotted time frame, specimen preservation is required.

1. 10% Formalin

Advantages

- Universal fixative.
- Simple to prepare and extended shelf life.
- The morphology of helminth eggs, larvae, protozoan cysts, and coccidia has been preserved well.
- Suitable for chromotrope, safranin, and acid-fast stains

Disadvantages

- Some permanent trichrome-stained smears are unsuitable.
- Inadequate preservation of the protozoan trophozoites' morphology.
- May disrupt PCR, especially after a prolonged fixation period.

2. Merthiolate-iodine-formaldehyde (MIF)

Advantages

- Components both fix and stain the organisms.
- Beneficial for field research.

Disadvantages

- Poor preservation of protozoan trophozoites morphology.
- Iodine interrupts fluorescence and other stains.

3. Low viscosity polyvinyl-alcohol (LV-PVA)

Advantages

- Protozoan trophozoites and cysts have their shape well preserved, and permanent smears stained with trichrome are simple to prepare.

Disadvantages

- Poor morphological preservation of helminth eggs, larvae, coccidia, and microsporidia.
- Not compatible with immunoassay kits.
- Unsuitable for chromotrope, safranin, and acid-fast stains.

4. Sodium acetate-acetic acid-formalin (SAF)

Advantages

- Both concentration processes and the preparation of permanently stained smears are suitable.

- Suitable for chromotrope, safranin and acid-fast stains.
- Suitable for use with immunoassay kits.

Disadvantages

- Adhesion of specimens on slides requires an additive, such as albumin-glycerin.
- Not as effective with permanent stains as PVA or Schaudinn's fixative.

Collection of Milk

Objective: For chemical examination in order to confirm mastitis.

Frequently, identifying the types of bacteria that are present in milk is required for controlling mastitis in animals. A milk sample taken from cows exhibiting clinical or subclinical mastitis symptoms must undergo a microbiological analysis, often known as a milk culture. The results of the milk cultures will aid in determining the specific bacteria responsible for the mastitis. This knowledge can then be applied to improve mastitis management, prevention, and treatment approaches to suit the needs of the herd.

Prior to administering antibiotics to the cow, milk samples must first be taken. Prior to milking, samples for culture should be taken. Individual samples should be taken from the afflicted quarters whenever there are clinical indications of mastitis or positive results from the California Mastitis Test. Composite samples (all four quarters in one collecting vial) will yield reasonable findings if the complete herd is being sampled.

Materials Required

- Nitrile or latex gloves
- Pre-dip (0.5% iodine or 4% hypochlorite)
- Cloth or paper towels
- Cotton balls that have been dipped in 70% ethyl or isopropyl alcohol
- Permanent marker
- Sterile pop-top or screw-on vials

Procedure

- Apply pre-dip to teats that have been cleared of manure, dirt, or sand while wearing clean gloves.
- Each teat should striped two to three streams of milk. The risk of contamination is decreased and the teat canal is flushed.

- With a separate paper or cloth towel, thoroughly dry each teat, paying close attention to the teat end.
- Wipe the end of the teat thoroughly with an alcohol-soaked cotton ball while keeping the top of the teat steady. Till the cotton ball still seems clean after use, use as many cotton balls as necessary.
- Without touching the inside of the tube or the bottom of the lid, open the milk vial and take a sample immediately. Fill the milk tube half to three-quarters full while holding the milk vial about 3 inches from the teat end.
- To stop dirt from falling into the vial, hold it at a 45° angle. When sampling, ensure not to place the teat inside the vial.
- As soon as possible, lock the lid and write the date, cow number, and sampled quarter on the top. Cool samples right away. Milk samples can be frozen for up to 6 months after being chilled for up to 2 days. Samples should be sent overnight on ice packs if being sent to a lab.
- Do not freeze the samples if users intend to ship them for somatic cell count examination because the cells will burst and an inaccurate reading will be obtained.

Preservation

- If milk is to be tested within a day or two (maximum 96 hours), the sample should be kept at **4°C.**
- If the sample needs to be preserved for a longer period of time, it must be stored at **-20°C.**

Collection of Synovial fluid

Objective: For diagnosis joint diseases.

Synovial fluid (SF) serves as a biological lubricant that reduces friction between the surfaces of the articular cartilage in synovial joints. It also serves as a source of nutrients for the tissues nearby and facilitates the movement of regulatory cytokines. As it is in close proximity to numerous tissues that are primarily altered during these disease processes, synovial fluid is of great interest for the investigation of orthopaedic pathologies, including osteoarthritis (OA), osteochondrosis, rheumatoid arthritis, and synovial sepsis, with minimally invasive collection protocols. Consequently, synovial fluid has the potential to enhance knowledge of the aetiology of underlying diseases and the discovery of biomarkers.

Site and Method

From affected joints, 5-10 ml from large animals (Cattle/Buffalo/Horse/ camels) and 0.5-1.0 ml from small animals (Dog, Cat, Sheep and goat)

- Anaesthetize with local anesthesia.
- Collect with an 18 gauze needle.
- Seal the joint with wound adhesive to prevent infection.

Preservation

- 3.8% sodium citrate (0.1 ml/ml of synovial fluid)
- EDTA
- Heparin

Collection of cerebrospinal fluid

Objective: Diagnosis of Central Nervous System (CNS) disorders.

CSF collection is an invasive technique that should only be carried out by trained professionals in an aseptic environment. The best clinical specimen to use for isolating, identifying, and characterisation of the etiological agents in cases of suspected bacterial meningitis is CSF. *Neisseria meningitidis*, *Streptococcus pneumoniae*, *Haemophilus influenzae*, and other pathogens might occasionally be considered as suspect agents.

Site

a) **Sub occipital region-**Horses, Sheep, Goats, Pigs and Dogs.

b) **Lumbosacral region-** Cattle and Buffaloes.

Methods

- Anesthetize the animal.
- Insert a 12 cm long needle with stylet in the mid line of soft depression between the dorsal process of lumbar vertebrae and the anterior end of median sacral crest, the point at the level of line joining anterior border of tuber coxae. The stylet is removed and the CSF is collected by syringe.

Preservation

For estimation of glucose, CSF should be collected in sodium fluoride. Other examination can be done without adding any preservative.

Collection of ascetic fluid and hydatid cyst fluid

Ascites fluid

The most frequent causes of ascites in pets: hypoproteinemia, left-sided heart failure, congestive heart failure, cirrhosis, hepatic illnesses, renal diseases, ancylostomosis, and bacterial infections like tuberculosis.

Abdominal paracentesis

- Disinfect the abdominal surface with 70% alcohol.
- Use 18-22 gauze sterile needles to allow good flow.
- Allow the ascites fluid to drip from the needle into a sterile collection tube.
- Allow to stand at Room Temperature for 30 min.
- Centrifuge to separate the serum (Straw coloured fluid) to sterile tube with a sterile syringe.

Preservation

Storage at – 70ºC.

Hydatid Cyst fluid

Hydatid cyst fluid (HCF), which fills the entire cyst, is a significant element of the interior environment. HCF is a liquid that is clear or clear yellowish and has antigenic qualities. HCF plays a significant part in the Echinococcus lifecycle by providing the nutrients required for larval growth.

- Aspirate by sterile needle in aseptic conditions.
- Centrifuge at 1000 rpm for 5 min, take the supernatant.

Preservation

Storage at -20ºC.

Specimen Labeling

All labeling needed to be done on specimen container. The other details of sender (name/address phone number) and test to be done from that sample labeled on the outer container.

Details of samples

- Animal species
- Breed

- Gender
- Age
- Date and Time of Collection
- Specimen ID

Documents to accompany

- A packing list or invoice form
- Air way bill (for travel by air) to be prepared by sender or shipper
- A value equivalence document (for land, rail, and maritime transportation)

Note

- An icebox or vaccination carrier can be used as an exterior container.
- The exterior container should have a minimum size of 10 x 10 x 10 cm (length x width x height).

Questions

1. Write the common anticoagulant and their use?
2. Difference between plasma and serum.
3. What preservative use to preserve urine, faeces and bacteriological samples?
4. Write the sites for collection of blood in cattle, pig, fowl and rat.

2

Clinical Significance and Interpretation of Serum Glucose

Rajesh Kumar Verma and Saurabh

Clinical Significance

The primary aim of laboratory diagnosis is to assess the carbohydrate metabolism impairment in diabetes mellitus, inducing the following:

1. Determination of glucose concentration in fasting blood and demonstration of postprandial glycosuria.
2. Assessment of glucose tolerance.

Interpretation

Hyperglycemia

Causes are:

1. **Diabetes mellitus**: Fasting blood sugar rise than normal. Values in uncertain range between these figures, calls for oral Glucose Tolerance Test to diagnose the condition.
2. **Hyperactivity of adrenal gland:** Hyperadrenocorticism (Cushing's disease) is a serious health condition in dogs that occurs when the adrenal glands overproduce cortisol (cortisone) in the animal's body. Excess cortisol can put a dog at risk of several serious conditions and illnesses, from kidney damage to diabetes, and can be life-threatening. Cortisol (also known as the stress hormone) is naturally produced in the body and is also found in certain medications. It can also happen because of certain medications that may be prescribed. Cushing's syndrome causes metabolic changes that make it more difficult for your body to regulate blood sugar. Cortisol hinders the effects of insulin in body. This results in an increased insulin resistance level.
3. **Pancreatic diseases:** Pancreatic diseases like Pancreatitis, cancer or cystic fibrosis, surgical removal of pancreas or haemachromatosis cause hyperglycemia. Diseases that are directly linked to pancreas can cause hyperglycemia. Pancreas is responsible for creating hormones and enzymes

for digestion, along with producing insulin. When animals or human body doesn't produce enough insulin, glucose is left to build up in bloodstream. That build-up of glucose is hyperglycemia.

4. **Obesity and Related Weight Factors:** Obesity is simply put an excessive amount of body fat. The condition can lead to inflammation, which can cause insulin resistance.
5. **Intracranial diseases:** Meningitis, encephalitis, tumors and hemorrhage show a moderate hyperglycemia.
6. **Lack of Physical Activity:** Physical activity is a vital part of maintaining a healthy body. When animal engage in physical activity, use energy stores. Energy is produced in the form of glucose by breaking down food into sugars. Physical activity makes the body more sensitive to insulin up to 24 hours after a workout. Even small amounts of exercise can help to prevent hyperglycemia.
7. **Polycystic Ovarian Syndrome:** Polycystic Ovarian Syndrome is a hormonal condition that affects female animals in their reproductive years, causing increased menstrual periods and high levels of androgen. Animal's ovaries may potentially release eggs in an irregular pattern as a result of this disease. Excess insulin is one of the causes of Polycystic Ovarian Syndrome. Excess insulin can develop to insulin resistance, which makes it difficult to control blood sugar levels.
8. **Trauma (Head Injury, Severe Burns, or Surgery):** Trauma to the body, or a severe injury, causes huge stress responses. Stress raises cortisol levels which lead to insulin resistance.
9. **Certain Medication:** Certain medications with steroids or diuretics can lead to higher blood glucose levels. Others can create insulin resistance.
10. **Diet (Excessive Amounts of Calories, Particularly Sugar/Carbohydrates):** The diet of animals plays a huge role in controlling blood sugar levels. This is important for diabetics and non-diabetics alike. Excessive sugar consumption in perpetuity can cause the body to cease responding to the insulin it produces. Over time, insulin resistance grows, and blood sugar levels continue to rise.

Hypoglycemia

When blood glucose falls below normal level.

1. Most commonly seen due to over dosage of insulin in treatment of diabetes mellitus.

2. Hypothyroidism- Cretinism, myxodema
3. Insulin secreting tumor of pancreas- rare
4. Hypoadrenalism (Addison's disease)
5. Hypopituitarism
6. Severe exercise.
7. Starvation

Along with estimation of blood glucose levels urine must be tested for

1. **Sugar-** Commonly in diabetes mellitus.
2. **Albumin-** Diabetic nephropathy
3. **Ketone bodies-** Diabetes ketoacidosis

Blood glucose level in animals

S. No.	Species	Blood glucose (mg/dl)
1.	Dog	60-110
2.	Cat	60-124
3.	Horse	62-114
4.	Cow	42-74
5.	Sheep	44-81
6.	Goat	48-76
7.	Pig	66-116

Glucose Tolerance Test

When the fasting blood sugar level is greater than 120 mg/dl (125 to 180 mg/dl), this test is used to confirm the diagnosis of diabetes mellitus. The concentration of blood glucose at defined intervals before and after the oral or intravenous administration of a given quantity of glucose is used to measure glucose tolerance. In dogs, both oral and intravenous approaches can be used. However, because there is no blood glucose response to oral glucose administration in ruminants, an intravenous approach must be used.

Oral method

After a 12-hour fast (if the animal is not hypoglycemic) and at appropriate intervals after administration, measure the glucose concentration. Orally administer 2.2 gram glucose/kg body weight to dogs. Give 1 gram glucose/kg body weight as a 20% solution through the stomach tube to the horse. Collect blood at an interval of 30 minutes for 3 to 4 hours or 6 hours (horses). The fasting sugar level in a normal dog is less than 120 mg/dl, does not exceed 160 mg/dl at the end of the first hour, and returns to normal at the end of the second hour. The fasting glucose level in a diabetic animal (dog) will be greater than 120 mg/dl; during the test, it will be greater than 180 mg/dl, and it will not return to normal during the 3 to 4-hour test.

Blood glucose levels in the horse reach approximately 175 mg/dl after 2 hours and return to baseline after 6 hours. Failure to return baseline values within the expected time frame may be interpreted as glucose intolerance, a feature of type 2 diabetes, hyperadrenocorticism, hypothyroidism, or hepatic insufficiency.

Intravenous method

After a 12-hour fast, inject 0.5 g/kg body weight of glucose as a 50% dog solution (not for ruminants) over a 30-second period and collect samples at 5, 15, 25, 35, 45, and 60 minutes. Plot the result on a log scale versus time and calculate the time required for the glucose value to decrease by half (normally 45 minutes or less in the dog). Long periods of disappearance indicate intolerance.

Sample required

Serum is the better option. If the plasma cannot be separated from the cells immediately, sodium fluoride is used. To obtain meaningful results, the sample must be properly collected and treated. Centrifuge the sample immediately, and then transfer the plasma or serum to another tube. If blood cells are allowed to remain in contact with serum or plasma, they will continue to use glucose at a rate of 7-10% per hour. Fasting samples are preferred (16-24 hours in dogs and cats). Fasting is not recommended for ruminants.

The following important types of response are seen commonly (dogs)

a) **Normal Response**: Fasting blood sugar is normal. After 1 hour level rises, but remain below the renal threshold of 180 mg/dl. It returns to normal fasting level within 2 hours.

b) **Diabetic curve**: Fasting level are (140 mg/dl) and 2 hour venous blood glucose of 200 mg/dl or more are diagnostic of diabetes. Glycosuria is unusually seen.

c) **Impaired GTT**: 2 hours values of blood glucose between 140 mg/dl and 200 mg/dl are not abnormal and must be followed up for DM.

d) **Renal Glycosuria**: Curve is normal. Due to lowered renal threshold one or more samples of urine contain glucose.

e) **Lag storage/ Alimentary Type**: Fasting blood glucose is normal. Due to rapid absorption, maximum levels may be reached at end of 2 hours.

f) **Flat curve of enhanced glucose tolerance**: the fasting blood glucose level is normal. Throughout the test the level does not vary + 20 mg%

Method of estimation

Nelson- Somogyi and ferricyanide methods: Reagents kits are also available.

The only sugar normally found in the blood is glucose, stored in the form of glycogen. Normally glycogen is found intracellular and the glucose extracellular. The level of blood glucose is maintained within a relatively narrow range, being controlled by several factors including hepatic and renal uptake and release of glucose, removal of glucose by peripheral tissue, hormonal influences on the processes and the absorption of glucose in the intestines (which has a temporary effect of blood glucose). The only sources of glucose are form liver and to a lesser extent kidney.

Questions

1. What is diabetic ketosis?
2. Define types of diabetes mellitus?
3. What are the main causes of hyperglycemic condition in animals?

3

Clinical Significance and Interpretation of Serum Protein

Saurabh

The liver produces the entire albumin and most of the globulin; a small amount of gamma globulin is produced by retculoendothelial tissue.

The production of albumin is subject to a mechanism regulating colloidal osmotic pressure and the secondary to alterations in globulin concentration. The liver synthesizes lipoproteins, glycoproteins, mucoproteins, fibrinogen, prothrombin and clotting factors VII, VIII, IX and X.

Total serum protein measurement is not directly indicative of the presence of any disease, but indirect correlation with disease process is extremely useful. Protein testing is recommended in cases of liver disease, immunosuppression, parasitic diseases, chronic wasting diseases, pregnancy, starvation, and edematous swelling of dependent body parts. Total proteins, albumin, globulin, albumin and globulin ration, and gamma globulin are all measured in serum.

Paper or cellulose electrophoresis allows fractionation and semiquantation of proteins in to 5 components, while the immunoelectrophoresis 30 or more components of serum protein can be separated.

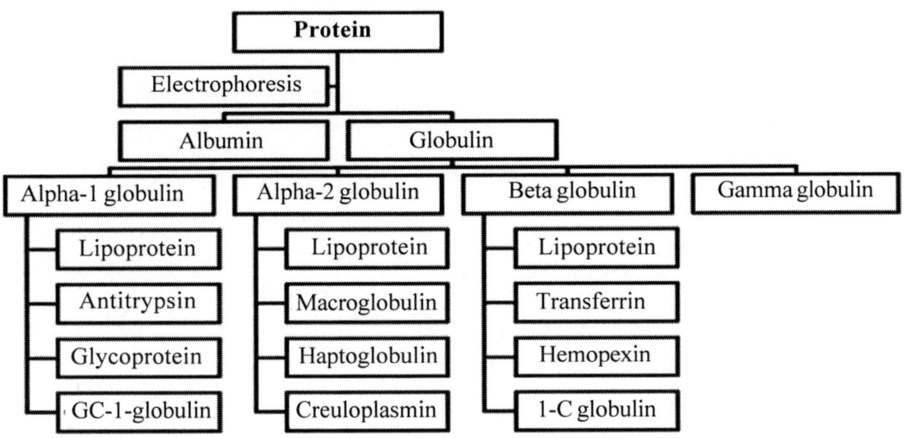

Fig. 1. Components of protein by electrophoresis method

Role of different types of proteins

a) **Lipoprotein**- These lipoproteins are essential for the small intestine to absorb and transport dietary lipids, for lipids to travel from the liver to peripheral tissues, and for lipids to travel from peripheral tissues to the liver and intestine (reverse cholesterol transport).

b) **Antitrypsin**- The liver produces alpha1-antitrypsin, a protein which provides protection to the lungs. A predisposition for obstructive lung disease and liver illness results from these proteins being deficient or malformed.

c) **Glycoprotein**- The structure, reproduction, immune system, hormones, and defense of cells and organisms are all regulated by glycoproteins. On the surface of cell membranes' lipid bilayers, glycoproteins can be seen.

d) **GC-1-globulin-** The main chemotactic enhancing factor in serum is GC-globulin, which has the potential to increase the chemotactic activity of peptides derived from C5.

e) **Macroglobulin**- In addition to regulating extracellular proteolysis, alpha-2-macroglobulin performs other tasks such directing proteolysis toward tiny substrates, promoting cell motility, and binding to cytokines, growth factors, and broken extracellular proteins.

f) **Haptoglobulin**- An acute phase protein called haptoglobulin has the ability to bind haemoglobin, reducing iron loss and kidney injury. Additionally, haptoglobin functions as an antioxidant, has antimicrobial properties, and affects many facets of the acute phase response.

g) **Creuloplasmin**- The protein ceruloplasmin is ferroxidase enzyme produced in the liver. Copper is transported and stored by it throughout the body. 65 to 90% of the copper in blood is transported by ceruloplasmin. Numerous bodily functions like iron metabolism depend on copper.

h) **Transferrin**- A blood-plasma glycoprotein called transferrin produces in liver is responsible for delivering ferric ions and is essential for iron metabolism. The most important ferric pool in the body is transferrin. It transports iron through the blood to various tissues such as the liver, spleen, and bone marrow.

Dysproteinemias

In order to interpret protein dyscrasias, we need to go for serum protein profile along with the A: G ratio in animals.

Procedure

- 3 test tubes should be placed on a test tube stand. Label the tubes with the letters "T" for test, "S" for standard, and "B" for blank. Pipette 4.9 mL of normal saline solution into tubes "T" and "S," and 5.0 mL into tube "B."
- Fill tube "T" with 0.1 mL test serum and tube "S" with 0.1 mL standard (0.4 percent bovine serum albumin in NSS).
- Add 5 mL of biuret reagent to each tube and thoroughly mix.
- Incubate the tubes in a 37°C water bath for 30 minutes.
- In a spectrophotometer, measure the absorbance or transmittance at 454 nm. Set zero to blank and use the following equation to calculate total serum protein:

Total serum protein (gram/100 ml)	= **OD of test / OD of standard**	**X Concentration of standard (gram/100 ml)**
....	....	....
....	....	....
....	....	....
....	....	....

Total Protein

Clinical Significance

Serum proteins vary widely in their size, structure and function. Abnormal levels of these proteins are terms dysproteinaemias. Total protein and albumin concentrations are determined and the globulin concentration arrived at by subtraction. Total protein levels are affected by physiological as well as pathological factors. Total protein levels are low in neonates rising to adult levels by 6 months to 1 year of age. In order animals total protein levels are high due mainly to IgG synthesis. Serum total protein levels are approximately 5% less than those of plasma due to the loss of fibrinogen in the clotting process.

Serum proteins in animals

S.No.	Animal species	Total protein (gm/dl)	Albumin (gm/dl)	Globulin (gm/dl)
1.	Dog	5.5- 7.5	2.6-4.0	2.1-3.7
2.	Cat	5.7- 8.0	2.4-3.7	2.4- 4.7
3.	Horse	5.7- 7.9	2.5-3.8	2.4-4.6
4.	Cow	6.2-8.2	2.8-3.9	2.9-4.9
5.	Sheep	5.9-7.8	2.7-3.7	3.2-5.0
6.	Pig	5.8-8.3	2.3-4.0	3.9-5.0
7.	Goat	6.1-7.4	2.3-3.6	2.7-4.4

Interpretation

The normal range of serum total proteins is 6-8 gm/100 ml. An increase in serum total proteins occurs in dehydration due to haemoconcentration. An increase may also occur in multiple myeloma, macroglobulinaemia, chronic infections, chronic liver disease and autoimmune disease and autoimmune diseases. A decrease in serum total proteins may results from heavy losses of proteins in urine as in nephritic syndrome. Protein under nutrition, intestinal malabsorption and protein losing enteropathy may also lower the serum total proteins. A decrease may also occur in shock, burns, crush injuries, haemorrhage etc. Due to haemodilution increased breakdown of proteins, as in hyperthyroidism, un-treated diabetes mellitus, wasting diseases etc. may also lower the level of proteins in serum.

Serum albumin

In conditions where the globulin level is to be calculated, albumin is measured in serum. The globulin content is calculated by subtracting the albumin values from the total serum proteins. The measurement of an albumin is indicated in all such situations in which total serum protein is determined.

The increase in serum albumin content is termed as hyperalbuminemia which is observed in shock, haemoconcentration, intestinal obstruction, severe burns, vomitions, diarrhea, hepatic disorder, chronic skin disease and acute dehydration. The hypoalbuminemia, decrease in albumin content in serum, is met in starvation, maldigestion, malabsorption, chronic hepatic diseases, prolonged fever, diabetes mellitus, acute nephritis, nephrosis, ascites, malnutrition, burns, candidiasis,

Serum globulin

Increase level of different types of globulin

Alpha globulin- alpha globulin level increases in serum analysis in acute and chronic renal disease, fever, destruction of tissue, in acute inflammatory process

Beta globulin- Increased levels of beta globulin occur in liver diseases, abnormal lipid metabolism like diabetes mellitus and hypothyroidism (beta globulin binds free and esterified cholesterol and phospholipids in serum), severe infection of helminthes in horses, chronic skin disease and eosinophilic myositis in dogs.

Gamma globulin- Level increases in new born animals, in response to high concentration of antigens, chronic inflammations like brucellosis and tuberculosis, in severe infectious diseases in bacterial, viral and parasitic infection, liver cirrhosis, equine infectious anaemia (albumin reduced).

Serum Albumin, Globulin, and A: G ratio

Clinical significance and interpretation

The normal range of serum albumin is 3.7-5.3 gm/100 ml Serum globulin ranges from 1.8 to 3.6 gm/100ml. the A: G ratio is roughly 2:1 through it may range from 1.2: 1 to 2.5:1. Decrease in serum albumin may occur in protein under nutrition, intestinal malabsorption, protein-losing enteropathy, liver disease, wasting diseases, nephritic syndrome and haemodilution. A severe decrease nephritic syndrome and haemodilution. A severe decrease or near-absence may be seen in an albuminaemia which is a genetic disease with autosomal recessive inheritance. A rise in serum albumin may occur in dehydration due to haemoconcentration. Serum globulin may decrease due to haemodilution in shock, burns, and haemorrhage etc. Serum globulin increases in multiple myeloma, macroglobulinaemia, chronic liver disease, chronic infections and autoimmune diseases. A: G ratio may be decreased or reversed in these conditions.

Questions

1. Which plasma protein is transporter of free fatty acids?
2. Name of plasma protein that binds extra corpuscular Hb?
3. What is analbuminemia?
4. What is meant by acute phase proteins? Acute phase of proteins are those proteins, the synthesis and thus the plasma level of which are increased in response to inflammation or tissue damage.
5. Which organ will be most affect when protein comes in urine.

4

Clinical Significance and Interpretation of Serum Lipid Profile and Serum Ketone Bodies

Saurabh

A. Triglycerides

Clinical significance

To form lipoproteins, triglycerides combine with cholesterol, phospholipids, and plasma proteins. To determine whether hypertriglyceridemia may be present, the serum triglyceride concentration is measured (increased blood and serum levels of triglycerides).

Chylomicrons and very low density lipoprotein (VLDLs), which cause the extensive lipaemia frequently observed in serum or plasma samples, are both mostly composed of glycerides.

An elevated level of serum triglycerides increases blood viscosity and precipitation, platelets aggregation which in turn results in diminished vascular flow. In addition, increased triglyceride concentrations in the blood coincide with decreased levels of HDL-cholesterol. Patients with ischemic vascular diseases frequently have elevated serum concentration of triglycerides.

Elevated levels

a) **Hypothyroidism**: Low amounts of "good" HDL cholesterol may result from it.
b) **Diabetes mellitus**: lowering triglyceride levels may help stave off diabetes, a serious condition that occurs when the body can't make the hormone insulin or use it well.
c) **Starvation**: The increased availability of free fatty acids during acute hunger is thought to be the cause of the rise in triglyceride content. Elevated secretin and glucagon levels are also thought to accelerate lipolysis and supply substrates for triglyceride synthesis.
d) **Hyperadrenocorticism:** Triglyceride and total cholesterol levels rise in hyperadrenocorticism, although HDL levels can fluctuate. Numerous

characteristics of the metabolic syndrome, such as insulin resistance, elevated fasting glucose levels, hypertension, obesity, and dyslipidemia, are shared by both overt and subclinical Hyperadrenocorticism.

e) **Biliary obstruction**- Serum Triglyceride and cholesterol level is elevated in cholestasis **because its metabolic degradation and excretion are impaired**. Bile is the normal excretory pathway for cholesterol and with reduced bile formation, cholesterol is retained.

f) **Pancreatitis**- Although rare, severe hypertriglyceridemia is a well-known cause of acute pancreatitis. Recent researches have revealed that persistent organ failure (POF) in acute pancreatitis is correlated with high blood triglyceride and low high-density lipoprotein cholesterol (HDL-C) levels.

g) **Glomerulopathy**- Increased triglycerides in chronic kidney disease (CKD) are caused by delayed degradation of triglyceride-rich lipoproteins, with no variations in production rate. Chronic kidney disease causes a down regulation of lipoprotein lipase and the LDL-receptor.

h) **Acromegally-** A pituitary adenoma-induced overproduction of growth hormone (GH) results in acromegaly. The lipid anomaly most frequently associated with acromegaly, hypertriglyceridemia, is likewise caused by GH-dependent inhibition of lipoprotein lipase function.

i) **Primary lipoproteinaemias**- Particularly, the transfer of triglycerides from chylomicrons and VLDL that are high in triglycerides to LDL is mediated by cholesterol ester transfer protein (CETP). Triglyceride content of LDL rises as a result of an increase in CETP-mediated exchange brought on by an increase in triglyceride-rich lipoproteins.

B. Cholesterol

Clinical Significance

Estimated of cholesterol is indicated in liver and thyroid dysfunction. The level of serum cholesterol is influenced by fat rich diet of animal containing saturated fatty acids.

Interpretation

Hypercholesterolemia causes- Nephritic syndrome, Hypothyroidism, Stress, High fat Diet, Bile duct obstruction, Leukemia Pregnancy, Nephritic syndrome.

Hypocholesterolemia causes-Hyperthyroidism Anaemia Hepatic disease Intestinal obstruction Polycythemia.

C. HDL-Cholesterol (Good Cholesterol)

Clinical significance

The main function of high density lipoproteins (HDL) is the transfer of cholesterol from peripheral tissues to the liver. HDL particles are mostly synthesized in the liver, and a minor part in intestinal cells. The nascent HDL particles contain phospholipids, cholesterol, Apo E and Apo A, and are discoid in shape. In the circulation, they assume a spherical shape due to the acceptance of Apo C and free cholesterol from other lipoproteins and non-fatty cells.

Interpretation

Determination of HDL-cholesterol is used in prevention diagnosis. Blood concentration of HDL-cholesterol is related with the occurrence of atherosclerotic disease, primarily coronary heart disease and peripheral circulation impairments. The lower blood concentration of HDL-cholesterol, the greater the risk of the disease.

D. LDL-Cholesterol (Bad Cholesterol)

Clinical Significance and Interpretation

LDL cholesterol testing is an important part of a CDH prevention strategy. It is used to further assess the risk of CDH when total cholesterol and /or HDL cholesterol results are abnormal. LDL cholesterol is used to monitor patients with prior CDH, other atherosclerotic disease, or diabetes mellitus.

Normal range of cholesterol

Animals	Normal Range of Cholesterol
Dog	115-250
Cat	90-130
Horse	70-145
Cow	80-120
Sheep	50-75
Pig	35-55
Goat	80-130

Clinical Significance and Interpretation of Ketone bodies

Ketone bodies (Acetone, Acetoacetic acid and β-hydrobutyric acid) are intermediary products of fat metabolism and their presence in the blood and then in the urine are indications that the metabolism is disordered or incomplete. This is associated with metabolic acidosis. This occurs in poorly controlled diabetes mellitus and also in starvation.

Ketosis of varying intensity, in fact, may occur in all mammalian species and can be brought forth, for example, by starvation, low carbohydrate and high fat diets, cold exposure, anesthesia, impaired liver function, hypoglycemia, and endocrine disorders such as diabetes or growth hormone and other endocrine excesses. Females of any species are more susceptible to ketosis than corresponding males, and this predisposition is exaggerated during lactation or pregnancy.

Exercise: to estimate serum ketones bodies and interpret from a clinical case.

Questions

1. Why density lipid (LDL) low is known as bad cholesterol?
2. What is triglycerides and their effect in body when increase in serum?
3. What are main causes of ketosis in animals?
4. Write the name of different ketone bodies.

5

Clinical Significance and Interpretation of Serum Minerals

Rajesh Kumar Verma

Calcium

Clinical Significance

Calcium is an essential mineral which is involved in many body systems. These include the skeleton, enzyme activation, muscle metabolism, blood coagulation and osmoregulation. In the blood calcium exists as 50% ionized, 40% protein bound and 10% complexes with anions such as citrate and phosphate. Only ionized calcium is biologically active in bone formation, neuromuscular activity, cellular biochemical processes and blood coagulation. Factors governing the total plasma concentration are complex and include interaction with other chemical moieties, proteins and hormones. Calcium, phosphorus and albumin metabolism are interdependent.

Interpretation

Elevated levels: (Hypercalcaemia)

a) **Lymphoproliferative disease (dogs)-** The release of parathyroid hormone-related peptide (PTHrP) by the tumour appears to be the most frequent cause of hypercalcemia linked to lymphomas.

b) **Hypoadrenocorticism (dogs)-** Electrolyte abnormalities, including mild to moderate hypercalcemia, may result from Hypoadrenocorticism.

c) **Malignant neoplasia-** The most frequent cause of hypercalcemia in malignancies is excessive parathyroid hormone-related peptide (PTHrP) production. It is also known by the name "humoral hypercalcemia of malignancy" (HHM).

d) **Primary renal failure (CRF or Familial)-** The hypercalcemia was caused by a combination of increased calcium input into the extracellular space and decreased calcium excretion by the kidney. Reduced glomerular filtration and higher tubular calcium reabsorption were the factors behind the decrease in calcium clearance.

e) **Primary hyperparathyroidism-** In primary hyperparathyroidism, the parathyroid glands enlarge, which results in an overproduction of parathyroid hormone which increases high blood calcium levels in the blood.

f) **Hypervitaminosis D-** Calcium levels in your blood can be elevated above normal by taking excessive vitamin D supplements over time.

Low level (Hypocalcaemia)

a) **Hypoalbuminae-** As a result of reduced calcium protein binding, hypoalbuminemia frequently coexists with hypocalcemia (as indicated by measurement of serum total calcium concentration).

b) **Malabsorption-** A case of severe hypocalcemia brought on by malabsorption as a result of small bowel Resection and partial gastrectomy.

c) **Acute pancreatitis-** Inflamed pancreas releases lipolytic products chelate calcium.

d) **Renal secondary hyperparathyroidism-** Vitamin D is not sufficiently converted by failing kidneys to its active form, and phosphate is not properly excreted. When this occurs, the body produces insoluble calcium phosphate, which removes calcium from the bloodstream. Both procedures result in secondary hyperparathyroidism and hypocalcemia.

e) **Primary hypoparathyroidism-** A rare endocrine condition called primary hypoparathyroidism is characterised by hypocalcemia as a result of the parathyroid glands' inability or failure to produce enough parathyroid hormone (PTH).

f) **Post thyroidectomy (cats)-** The thyroid gland secretes thyrocalcitonin (TCT), which regulates blood calcium levels.

g) **Ethylene glycol poisoning-** Oxalic acid is the last product of the metabolism of ethylene glycol. Oxalic acid and calcium bind very readily, resulting in the characteristic urine oxalate crystals. Systemic hypocalcemia may occur if calcium is consumed after complexing with oxalate.

h) **Glucocorticoid therapy-** Numerous pathways exist for how steroids promote bone loss. They have the effect of reducing intestinal calcium absorption and raising urine calcium loss.

Phosphorus (Inorganic Phosphate)

Clinical Significance

Serum phosphorus is primarily regulated by the kidney through the action of parathyroid hormone. Abnormal levels are caused by variations in dietary intake, decreased renal excretion and the hormonal imbalances that affect serum calcium.

Interpretation

Elevated level: Prerenal, renal & post renal azotemia, Young animals (<1 yr), Hyperthyroidism, Secondary Hyperparathyroidism, Primary Hypoparathyroidism, Hypervitaminosis D, Tissue necrosis, Osseous Neoplasia

Low level: Malignant neoplasia, Glucocorticoid therapy, Primary Hyperparathyroidism, Oral phosphate-binding agents, Osteomalacia, Hyperadrenocorticism, Hypovitaminosis D, Renal tubular defects

Prerenal, renal and post renal azotemia- Extra phosphorus is removed from the blood by healthy kidneys. Insufficient kidney function can result in a high blood phosphorus level, which increases your risk of heart disease, weak bones, joint pain, and even death.

Young animals (<1 yr)- Young and growing animals exhibit physiologically raised serum and plasma phosphorus concentrations as a result of increased intestinal phosphorus intake and decreased renal phosphorus excretion, likely to promote bone mineralization.

Secondary Hyperparathyroidism- The most frequent cause of secondary hyperparathyroidism is chronic renal failure. Vitamin D is not sufficiently converted by failing kidneys to its active form, and phosphate is not properly excreted. When this occurs, the body produces insoluble calcium phosphate, which removes calcium from the bloodstream.

Hypervitaminosis D- By facilitating Calcium and Phosphorus absorption from the kidneys and intestines, vitamin D helps to maintain the body's calcium (Ca) and phosphorus (P) balance. Level of Ca and P absorption increases in hypervitaminosis D condition.

Normal range of Calcium and Phosphorus in blood

Minerals	Dog	Cat	Horse	Cattle	Sheep	Pig	Goat
Calcium (mg/dl)	8.7-11.8	7.9-10.9	10.4-13.4	8.4-11.0	9.3-11.7	9.3-11.5	9-11.6
Phosphorus (mg/dl)	3.0-6.2	4-7.3	2.3-5.4	4.3-7.8	4-7.3	5.5-9.3	3.7-9.7

Questions

1. Role of calcium in animal body
2. Role of phosphorus in animal body

6

Clinical Significance and Interpretation of Serum Electrolytes

Rajesh Kumar Verma

Sodium

Clinical Significance

Compared to potassium, sodium is distributed differently throughout the body. Due to the sodium pump mechanism, most sodium is extracellular. Compared to this, just 2% of potassium is extracellular; the remainder is intracellular. Regarding the plasma concentrations of sodium and potassium, renal function is the single most significant homeostatic mechanism.

Small animals frequently experience mild hyponatraemia. A significant hyponatraemia or a sodium to potassium ratio of less than 27:1 calls for additional research. A marked hyponatremia may result in fluid entering cells, which might affect the nervous system functions. Small animals rarely get hypernatraemia. It almost invariably means that the amount of water being consumed is insufficient to offset fluid loss. Due to the net migration of water out of the cells, marked hypernatraemia may cause neurological symptoms.

The levels of sodium in the extracellular fluid are a reflection of the proportions of water and electrolytes. It is the key factor in determining ECF volume. More frequently than because of decreased intake, hyponatraemia is caused by excessive losses. A water loss that exceeds electrolyte loss is hypernatraemia.

Interpretation

Elevated levels (Hypernatraemia) causes- Diabetes mellitus, Diabetes insipidus, Hyperadrenocorticism, Increased sodium intake, Moderate dehydration, Pyometra, Osmotic diuresis, Osmotic cathartics, Water restriction, Extreme exercise, Drug therapy (e.g.corticosteroids), Severe hypokalaemia

a) **Diabetes mellitus**- An osmotic force generated by higher glucose concentration pulls water into the extracellular space. As a result, plasma sodium levels are reduced and extracellular sodium is diluted.

b) **Diabetes insipidus-** A diagnosis of diabetes insipidus can be made based on certain blood and urine tests, including those that reveal low urine concentration, hypernatraemia (high blood salt levels), and serum or plasma osmolality (high blood concentrations) (urine osmolality).

c) **Hyperadrenocorticism-** Recent research suggests that ACTH can boost the adrenal cortex's ability to regulate salt levels, which in turn reduces sodium and increases potassium excretion in the urine. The sodium ion concentration decreases in sweat. As a result, blood sodium levels rise.

d) **Moderate dehydration-** When an individual excretes too much water without also excreting electrolytes, it leads to hypertonic dehydration, which results in extracellular fluid (the fluid that surrounds cells) having a high sodium concentration. When sodium is present in large quantities outside of a cell, water is drawn away from the cell and toward the sodium.

e) **Pyometra-** Pyometra causes dehydration so sodium ion concentration increases in serum.

f) **Osmotic diuresis-** The total loss of sodium and potassium per litre of urine during osmotic diuresis is less than the concomitant serum sodium level. As a result, hypernatremia may develop.

g) **Osmotic cathartics-** An Osmotic cathartic increases the water content and weight of the feces using the principle of osmosis into gastrointestinal tract or GIT. Dehydration occurs and may develop hypernatremia.

h) **Water restriction-** Limiting water intake rapidly raises the plasma sodium as the excess water is readily excreted.

i) **Extreme exercise-** Excessive sweating by exercise and other extrarenal forms of water loss induce some sodium loss, but because sweat is hypotonic (especially in animals that have acclimated to the heat), severe hypovolemia can occur before significant hypovolemia.

j) **Drug therapy (e.g.corticosteroids)-** Corticosteroids. Prednisone is one of many corticosteroid medications that can result in sodium retention and dose-related fluid retention. The most fluid retention is brought on by corticosteroids with potent mineralocorticoid effects, such as hydrocortisone and fludrocortisone.

k) **Severe hypokalaemia-** When the body is depleted of potassium, cells must take up sodium from the extracellular fluid in order to maintain volume and tonicity. This leads to hyponatremia and hypokalemia. Depletion of potassium also encourages renal salt retention, which raises exchangeable sodium.

Low levels (Hyponatraemia) causes

Hypoadrenocorticism, Severe dehydration (vomiting and diarrhea), Certain medications (Diuretics, Pain killer and antidepressants), Problems with the heart, kidneys, and liver, Inappropriate anti-diuretic hormone (SIADH) Syndrome,

Hormonal changes

a) **Hypoadrenocorticism:** Animals with adrenal insufficiency frequently experience hyponatremia, which is brought on by an inappropriate rise in vasopressin secretion or activity as a result of low cortisol levels and an inability to eliminate free water.

b) **Severe dehydration (vomiting and diarrhea):** This raises levels of ADH while also causing the body to lose electrolytes like sodium.

c) **Certain medications (Diuretics, Pain killer and antidepressants):** Various drugs, such as some diuretics (water pills), pain relievers, and antidepressants, can disrupt the hormonal and kidney functions that regulate salt levels within a healthy normal range.

d) **Problems with the heart, kidneys, and liver:** Congestive heart failure and some disorders of the kidneys or liver can lead to fluid accumulation in the body, which dilutes the sodium in the body and lowers the overall amount.

e) **Inappropriate anti-diuretic hormone (SIADH) Syndrome:** When this condition develops, the body produces excessive amounts of the anti-diuretic hormone (ADH), which prevents the body from excreting water normally through urination.

f) **Hormonal changes:** Adrenal gland insufficiency reduces the adrenal glands' capacity to generate hormones that support the body's sodium, potassium, and water balance. Low blood sodium levels can also be brought on by low thyroid hormone levels.

Potassium

Clinical Significance

Plasma potassium levels are not always a good indicator of intracellular levels; in acidosis the exchange of H^+ and K^+ ions leads to the depletion of intracellular potassium and elevated plasma potassium. The converse occurs in alkalosis. Hypokalaemia may lead to neurological, muscular and cardiac signs. In most cases, hyperkalaemia arises due to a diminished ability to excrete potassium. Marked hyperkaelaemia is potentially life threatening causing bradycardia and cardiac arrest.

Interpretation

Elevated level (Hyperkalaemia): Acute renal failure, A diet high in potassium, Drug action, Hypoadrenocorticism, Burns or severe injuries, Poorly controlled diabetes, Metabolic acidosis, Urethral obstruction, Bladder rupture

Low level (Hypokalaemia): Diuretic therapy, Diabetes mellitus, Polyuric disorders, Vomiting and diarrhea, Chronic renal failure (particularly cats), Insulin therapy, Steroid administration, Excessive bicarbonate therapy, Administration of potassium depleted fluid, Excessive mineralocorticoid therapy

Elevated level (Hyperkalaemia)

a) **Acute renal failure:** Hyperkalemia can occur if the kidneys are not functioning properly. The kidneys' task is to maintain a balance between the potassium consumed and the potassium lost in urine. Animals consume potassium by eating certain meals. It is excreted through urine after being filtered by the kidneys. High potassium levels are frequently compensated for by the kidneys in the early stages of renal disease. However, when the kidneys' ability to filter out potassium from your body declines, they might not be able to do so. Hyperkalemia frequently results from advanced renal disease.

b) **A diet high in potassium:** Eating too many foods high in potassium can also lead to hyperkalemia, particularly in those with advanced kidney disease. Bananas, orange juice, cantaloupe, honeydew melon, and other foods are rich in potassium.

c) **Drug action:** Medications that stop the kidneys from sufficiently losing potassium. Certain medications may prevent the kidneys from excreting adequate potassium. The potassium levels may increase as a result.

d) **Hypoadrenocorticism:** In primary hypoadrenocorticism, aldosterone deficit leads the kidneys to fail to retain salt and eliminate potassium, which results in hyperkalemia and hyponatremia.

e) **Burns or severe injuries:** This happens as a result of the body releasing additional potassium into the blood in reaction to severe burns or wounds.

f) **Poorly controlled diabetes:** Hyperkalemia refers to an excess of potassium. Animals and humans with poorly controlled diabetes may experience this issue. The kidneys, which typically eliminate excess potassium from the body, are damaged by high blood sugar. Heart issues and other consequences are more prevalent in those with diabetes and high potassium levels.

g) **Metabolic acidosis:** In metabolic acidosis condition hydrogen ions (H^+) and potassium ion (K^+) pump activate, the potassium ion comes into blood and hydrogen ions goes into cells to compensate acidosis.

h) **Urethral obstruction:** Complete lower urinary tract obstruction is more likely to result in hyperkalemia and severe metabolic acidosis than postrenal azotemia.

i) **Bladder rupture:** An intraperitoneal bladder rupture in animals who have gastrointestinal symptoms and indications, haematuria, and the biochemical indicators are elevated serum urea, creatinine, and potassium, reduced serum sodium, and CO_2 content.

Low level (Hypokalaemia)

Diuretic therapy, Diabetes mellitus, Polyuric disorders, Vomiting and diarrhea, Chronic renal failure (particularly cats), Insulin therapy, Excessive bicarbonate therapy, Excessive mineralocorticoid therapy

a) **Diuretic therapy**- Too much potassium may be excreted through the urine when taking diuretics.

b) **Vomiting and diarrhea**- Vomiting, diarrhea or both also can result in excessive potassium loss from the digestive tract.

c) **Diabetes mellitus**- Among the factors that contribute to hypokalemia in diabetics are: (1) redistribution of potassium [K+] from the extracellular to the intracellular fluid compartment (shift hypokalemia brought on by insulin administration); (2) gastrointestinal loss of K+ as a result of malabsorption syndromes (diabetic-induced motility disorders, bacterial overgrowth, chronic diarrheal states); and (3) renal loss of K+ as a result of osmotic diuresis.

d) **Chronic renal failure (particularly cats)**- There is currently little knowledge of the precise mechanism causing significant hypokalemia in feline CKD patients. It is probably caused by a combination of increased urine loss brought on by polyuria, which leaves less room for reabsorption, low food intake, renin-angiotensin-aldosterone system activation.

e) **Insulin therapy**- Treatment with insulin decreases K+ levels, causing K+ to enter cells (both directly and indirectly by reversing hyperglycemia). As a result, insulin therapy has the potential to result in severe hypokalemia, especially in animals or humans who had normal or low serum K+ content at the time of presentation.

f) **Excessive mineralocorticoid therapy**- Potassium loss may have been caused by an excess of mineralocorticoids brought on by the use of anabolic steroids, together with a high carbohydrate/hypercaloric load that resulted in an influx of intracellular potassium through the action of insulin and resultant severe hypokalemia.

g) **Excessive bicarbonate therapy**- Lowers potassium ion.

Chloride

Chloride is present in highest concentrations in the ECF and tends to accompany sodium movement by passive diffusion.

Interpretation

Elevated levels (Hyperchloraemia): Dehydration, Acidosis, Respiratory alkalosis, Renal dysfunction

Low levels (Hypochloraemia): Gastro-intestinal loss (high bowl obstruction), Low salt diet, Respiratory acidosis, Oesophageal obstruction.

Elevated levels (Hyperchloraemia)

There are numerous circumstances that could lead to hyperchloremia. The first situation is when electrolyte-free fluid is lost. This simply implies that the body is shedding more fluids which do not contain electrolytes, like chloride, leading to a high concentration of these ions in the body. This fluid loss can be brought on by sweating (due to activity or temperature), skin burns, dehydration, a hypermetabolic condition, or diabetes insipidus. Feelings of dehydration and dry mucous membranes might result from fluid loss.

The second scenario, known as loss of hypotonic fluid, which can be a direct result of electrolyte fluid loss, may result in hyperchloremia. In the body, water typically moves from a region with low ion concentration to one with a high ion concentration. Less water is available to diluted these high ion concentration locations in this situation since the water is being expelled in the urine. This may be brought on by the use of diuretics, vomiting, diarrhoea, burns, kidney disease, kidney failure, and acidity of the renal tubules. Additionally, this could cause you to feel dehydrated.

An increase in the intake of sodium chloride is the third situation that could result in hyperchloremia. Dietary intake or intravenous fluid administration in a medical context may be to blame for this. Hypertension, edoema, and cardiovascular dysfunction may result from this.

Low levels (Hypochloraemia)

Loss of gastric contents usually results in excessive loss of chloride (high bowl obstruction). As a result of increased renal excretion of chloride together with potassium and ammonium, the low serum chloride that results from respiratory acidosis is instead accompanied by a net loss of chloride from the body. In particular, prolonged vomiting may deplete chloride to a higher degree than sodium due to the high proportion of chloride in gastric fluid.

Normal range of electrolytes in serum

Electrolytes	Dog	Cat	Horse	Cattle	Sheep	Pig	Goat
Sodium (mEq/L)	140-153	145-159	133-147	134-148	141-160	139-160	136-152
Potassium (mEq/L)	3.9-5.6	3.8-5.3	2.8-4.7	4-5.8	4.3-6.3	4.4-6.5	3.8-5.7
Chloride (mEq/L)	102-117	107-130	97-110	96-109	100-113	97-107	100-112

Questions

1. Write name of chief extracellular cation and anion in animals
2. Write intracellular cation and anion in animals
3. Write cause of hypernatraemia in animals.

7

Clinical Significance and Interpretation of Serum Creatinine, Urea (Bun) and Uric Acid

Rajesh Kumar Verma

Creatinine

Clinical significance

Creatinine is produced at a steady rate due to muscle catabolism and is not reabsorbed by the kidney tubules after filtration. Its measurement provides an indirect assessment of the glomerular filtration rate (GFR). Unlike urea it is not markedly affected by diet or any aspect of liver function and therefore the test is more specific for renal dysfunction.

Interpretation

Elevated levels

a) Renal, pre renal and post renal Azotaemia-

Renal

i) A kidney infection

ii) **Glomerulonephritis**, which is inflammation of the kidney structures that filter the blood

iii) **Kidney failure**

Prerenal

i) Haemorrhage

ii) Shock

Post renal

i) Leakage in urinary tract

ii) Blockage of urinary tract by Kidney stone

b) Severe prolonged excretion or exercise

c) Acute myositis or muscle trauma

d) Cooked meat diet

e) Increase pituitary activity

f) Placental dysfunction

The blood creatinine is kept in a normal range by the kidneys. The kidney's ability to function is generally indicated by creatinine. A high creatinine level indicates either renal disease or reduced kidney function.

The blood level of creatinine will increase if the kidneys become impaired for any reason because the kidneys are unable to adequately remove creatinine from the body. Thus, abnormally high creatinine levels serve as a warning sign for potential renal damage or failure. Because of this, normal blood tests assess the blood's level of creatinine on a regular basis.

The amount of creatinine removed from the body by the kidneys can be calculated to get a more accurate estimate of renal function. This measures the rate of filtration by the kidneys and is known as creatinine clearance (glomerular filtration rate or GFR).

Urea

Clinical significance

The liver's process of determining amino acids mostly results in urea. Urea is created when nitrogen content of ammonia, mixes with other components like carbon, hydrogen, and oxygen. The bloodstream carries urea, a chemical waste product, from the liver to the kidneys. This urea is filtered by healthy kidneys, which also eliminate other blood waste products from urine. The most common test for renal function is urea, which is mainly produced exerted by the kidneys.

Interpretation

Elevated levels- Renal azotaemia, Acute renal failure, Chronic renal failure, Pre renal azotaemia, Shock, High protein diet, Fever, Reduced cardiac output, Hyperthyroidism (cats), Hypoadrenocorticism, Gastrointestinal haemorrhage, Prolonged exercise, Corticosteroid therapy, Post renal Azotaemia, Feline urological syndrome, Bladder rupture, Calculi, Neoplasia Perineal herniation

Low level- Polydipsia/ polyuria, Hepatic insufficiency, Protein malnutrition, Over hydration, Late pregnancy, Anabolic steroids

Blood Urea Nitrogen

BUN is measure of the amount of nitrogen in the blood in the form of urea and a measurement of renal function.

Urea = BUN X 2.14

Mol. Wt of Urea = 60

Urea Nitrogen = 28

Factor = 60/28 = 2.14

A high BUN level typically indicates that your kidneys aren't functioning properly. Elevated BUN, however, can also result from:

i) Dehydration due to inadequate fluid intake or for other reasons
ii) Blockage of the urinary tract
iii) Recent heart attack or congestive heart failure
iv) Bleeding from the gut
v) Shock
vi) Severe burns
vii) Several drugs, including several antibiotics
viii) A diet rich in protein

Uric Acid

A typical bodily waste product is uric acid and a form by the breakdown of chemical purines. The body naturally contains chemical called purines. Additionally, purines can be present in a variety of foods like liver, seafood, and alcohol. Purines can also be formed when DNA is broken down in the body.

Clinical significance and interpretation

Increased levels of uric acid are associated with gout, renal failure and large dietary intake of purines.

A high uric acid level typically results from ineffective uric acid elimination by your kidneys. Rich meals, being overweight, having diabetes, taking some diuretics (also known as water pills), consuming excessive amounts of alcohol, and having diabetes are all factors that could contribute to this slowing down of uric acid clearance.

Normal range of creatinine and Blood urea nitrogen (BUN)

Electrolytes	Dog	Cat	Horse	Cattle	Sheep	Pig	Goat
Creatinine (mg/dl)	0.5-1.6	0.5-1.9	0.9-2.0	0.6-1.8	0.9-2.0	0.8-2.3	0.7-1.5
Blood urea nitrogen (mg/dl)	8.8-25.9	15.4-31.2	10.4-24.7	7.8-24.6	10.3-26.0	8.2-24.6	12.6-25.8

Questions

1. Define types of azotemia?
2. Define role of Creatinine in kidney function test?
3. In initial stage of renal dysfunction, which test is more sensitive?

8

Urine Examination Clinical Significance and Interpretation

Saurabh

Urinnalysis

An essential laboratory test that is easily conducted in veterinary settings and is included in a basic database is urinalysis. Documenting diverse urogenital tract conditions is helpful, because it could reveal details about other systemic conditions including hemolysis and liver failure. Cystocentesis, urethral catheterization, or simply voiding can all be used to collect urine. Urine should be examined within 30 minutes, but if this is not possible, it can be refrigerated for up to 24 hours or sent to a outside diagnostic lab; this, however, may cause crystal precipitation. The pH or specific gravity of urine are unaffected by refrigeration. Preservative should be added if cytologic analysis is necessary and a delay in slide preparation is anticipated. A few drops of 10% formalin (exact concentration not necessary) are better than boric acid.

Methods of urine collection

For the collection of urine, the container (glass vials or disposable plastic container) must be clean. If quick examination is not possible, use opaque plastic or dark glass to stop the degradation of constituents like bilirubin and urobilinogen that are sensitive to sunlight.

There are three methods for the urine collection

a) **Cystocentesis:** Urine is drawn from the bladder using a syringe and sterilised needle. Urine is taken directly into the sterile syringe after the needle is inserted through the abdominal wall into a full bladder. The benefit of cystocentesis is that no other debris from the lower urinary tract is present to contaminate the urine. This kind of sample is excellent for evaluating the kidneys and bladder as well as for identifying bacterial infections. Cystocentesis has a few drawbacks, including the fact that it is a little more invasive than other techniques that it is only effective when the pet's bladder is full, and that it can be challenging to perform on uncooperative pets.

b) **Catheterization:** The lower urinary tube, often known as the urethra, is used to insert a very narrow, sterile catheter into the bladder. Urine is taken from the bladder into a sterile syringe that is connected to the catheter. When a voluntary sample is not available, the method-which is less invasive than cystocentesis-is a suitable choice, particularly in male dogs. The urethra has only minor irritation as a result of catheterization, and the germs there may enter the bladder from the urethra.

c) **Mid-stream free flow:** Pets voluntarily urinate as usual, and as they do so, a sample is taken and placed in a sterile container. The sample should ideally be taken mid-stream, or halfway through urinating. The terms "free flow" and "free catch" are frequently used to describe this kind of sample. This approach has the benefits of being fully non-invasive and allowing the pet owner to collect the urine sample at home. The drawbacks include the potential difficulty of taking a sample mid-stream from some pets and the increased risk of environmental or urethral debris contaminating the urine.

Preservatives

Preservatives may be used when immediate analysis or refrigeration is not possible.

S. No.	Preservatives	Advantages	Disadvantages	Additional information
1.	**Refrigeration**	Does not interfere with chemical test	Precipitates amorphous phosphates & urates	Prevents bacterial growth for 24 hour
2.	**Thymol**	Antimicrobial	A false positive protein reaction will result with sulfosalicylic acid method	Often combines with sodium fluoride to preserve glucose
3.	**Taluene**	Antimicrobial, does not interfere with chemical determination of protein or glucose	Changes the amount of ketones	Useful to preserve a 24 hr urine specimen obtained in a metabolic cage
4.	**Formalin (Formaldehyde)**	Prevents bacterial growth, excellent sediment (casts and cellular elements)	Interfere with glucose, blood, leukocyte esterase & copper reduction	One drop of 40% formalin in 30 ml of urine preserve cast & cellular elements
5.	**Boric acid**	Prevents bacterial growth and metabolism (antimicrobial)	-	Used when hormones analysis of specimen is required

6.	**Chloroform**	Antibacterial	-	5 ml is sufficient to preserve 24 hr urine collection
7.	**Sodium fluoride**	Good preservative for drug analysis	Inhibit reagent strip tests for glucose, blood and leukocytes	-
8.	**Metaphosphoric acid**	Preservative for vitamin C (ascorbic acid)	-	1 volume of aq 10% conc. Is added to 5 volume of urine for analysis of Vitamin- C

Urine examination

A fresh sample is preferred for the analysis of urine. If urine is contaminated by urea-splitting bacteria, which are often found in the urethra, it may lose its diagnostic value if it is left to stand for several hours at room temperature because urea splits into ammonia and urine becomes alkaline.

A. Physical examination

Interpretation

a) **Volume**: The amount of volume produced per day depend variables like diet, fluid intake, climate, exercise, size and body weight. Urine volume is inversely proportional to specific gravity except in diabetes mellitus (high volume and increased specific gravity due to glycosuria).

Polyuria (increased volume)	Oliguria (Decreased volume)
Nephritis	Fever
Diabetes mellitus	Shock
Diabetes insipidus	Acute renal failure
General liver disease	Heart disease
Pyometra	dehydration

b) **Appearance/colour:** On visual inspection, normal urine is often transparent and yellow or amber in colour. It is important to consider urine specific gravity when interpreting the colour since it is partly influenced by the amount of urine that was collected and the concentration of urine that was produced. Even when the urine is normal in colour, severe diseases may still persist. Although it doesn't give precise information, abnormal urine colour may be produced by the presence of endogenous or exogenous pigments. The yellow color of concentration urine is due to "urochrome".

Colour of urine	Causes
Clear, very pale straw colour	Low specific gravity (dil. Urine)
Clear to slightly turbid, deep yellow	High specific gravity (conc. Urine)
Amber urine	Conjugated bilirubin
Red urine	Hemoglobin (blood, free), myoglobin, porphyria, drugs (phenolphthalein, deferoxamine, some phenothiazines
Red-pink	Consumption of beetroot or red food dyes
Smoky/ brown urine	Altered blood (acid hematin), alkaptonuria (turns brown on standing), melanin (i.e., disseminated melanoma)
Dark orange urine	Drugs (pyridium, rifampin, others).
Fluorescent yellow	Vitamins
Foamy urin	Proteinuria, conjugated bilirubin.
Turbid/ cloudy urine	WBC's, urates, phosphates cells, RBC, Epithelial cells, casts, ,Mucus, Bacteria, Amorphous material crystals
Fat globules on surface	Fat embolization

c) **Odour**: The ammonia odour of typical urine varies depending on urine content. Some species, like cats and goats, have pungent urine odor because of the composition of their urine. A bacterial infection may cause a strong odour because of pyuria; if the bacteria produce urease, a strong ammonia odour may happen. Volatile organic acids are the cause of the typical odour. Free degraded urine produces an ammoniac odour as a result of urea decomposition. A sweetish, fruity odour is produced when ketone bodies are present. The excretion of some medications gives a distinctive odour. When urine is kept at room temperature for an extended period of time or when cystitis is present, excessive urine breakdown by bacteria causes an abnormally foul odour.

Turbidity

Although urine is normally clear, conditions like pigmenturia, crystalluria, hematuria, pyuria, lipiduria, or the presence of other substances like mucus may cause it to become less transparent. Depending on the cause, the sample's increased turbidity may go away after centrifugation.

Specific gravity

With the use of a urinometer created with veterinary samples, the Urine Specific Gravity (USG) is calculated. USG in healthy animals varies greatly depending on the body's fluid and electrolyte balance. Therefore, the clinical presentation and serum chemistry results must be considered while interpreting a USG. An animal with prerenal azotemia from dehydration or other reasons will have hypersthenuric urine with a USG > 1.025-1.040 (Depending on species). It is abnormal for an animal that is dehydrated or azotemic to have dilute urine, which can be brought on by renal failure, hypo- or hyperadrenocorticism, hypercalcemia, diabetes mellitus diuretic treatment, hyperthyroidism, or diabetes insipidus. Despite increased urine volume, an elevated USG is the result of glucoseuria increasing the urine's refractive index.

Alternation in urine specific gravity and their causes

Specific gravity	Clinical finding	Causes
>1.030 dog>1.035 cat	Dehydration	Increased water relation by the kidney causes hyperosmolarity
<1.030 dog<1.035 cat	Dehydration	Renal concentrating deficiency brought on by extra renal or renal illness
1.012-1.030 dog 1.012-1.035 cat	Polyuria	Acute renal failure
1.020-1.030	Polyuria/Polydipsia	Diabetes mellitus, Hyperadrenocorticism
1.008-1.012	Polyuria/Polydipsia	With Oliguria: acute renal failureWith polyuria: chronic renal failure, post-urinary obstruction
1.008-1.012Or <1.008	Polyuria/Polydipsia (with no azotemia)	**Calcium**- Hypercalcaemia
		Cholesterol, Alkaline phosphatase (ALP), glucose-Hyperadrenocorticism, steroid therapy
		Inflammatory leucogram- pyelonephritis, Pyometra
		Na^+ and K^{+-}- Hypoadrenocorticism
		T 4- Hyperthyroidism (cats)
		bile acids- Hepatic insufficiency
<1.008	Polyuria/ Polydipsia	Central or nephrogenic diabetes insipidus

Differentiation of common causes of altered urine gravity

Condition	Specific Gravity
Usual range in healthy dogs Usual range in healthy cats	1.015- 1.0451.035- 1.060
Possible range	1.001-1.080
Hyposthenuria	<1.008-1.012
Isosthenuria	1.008-1.012
Hyperstenuria	>1.012

f) **Urine pH:** For both dogs and cats, the normal urine pH range is 6 to 7.5. Urine pH can be impacted by an illness patient's acid-base balance. Because the kidneys neutralize the consequences of a pH change in the body, systemic acid-base imbalances alter the pH of the urine. Urinary tract infections caused by bacteria that produce urease (which converts urea to ammonia) might result in an increase in urine pH (alkaline urine). If a dog or cat has alkaline urine, it should be examined to see if white cells or bacteria are presented (often evident in urine sediment). Diets high in animal protein (usually ingested by dogs and cats) produce a lower urine pH (acidic urine).

Higher urine pH is a result of plant- or vegetable-based diets (usually ingested by ruminants and horses) (alkaline urine). Animals fed milk-based diets tend to have acidic urine. Urine pH can rise when samples are not quickly evaluated. For example, when carbon dioxide diffuses into the atmosphere from the urine, the pH rises because carbon dioxide behaves as an acid.

Because some crystals, like struvite, form in alkaline urine while others, like cystine, do in acidic urine, urine pH will have an impact on crystalluria.

B. Chemical examination

a) Protein

Proteins are coagulated by strong acids and alkaloid reagents. Test for proteins is done by using this property of protein.

i) **Sulphosalicylic acid test:** Fill a test tube with 2.0 ml of sulphosalicylic acid. Add urine drop by drop to keep the two layers apart. The presence of protein is shown by the development of a white precipitation ring at the junction of two layers. When the two layers are mixed, the entire solution turns turbid, confirming the presence of protein in the urine.

ii) Heller's ring test: Fill the test tube with 3.0 ml of concentrated HNO3 (nitric acid). Add 3.0 ml of urine into a test tube such that the both liquids do not mix. The presence of protein is shown by the white ring's appearance.

Clinical significance: Albumin, which has passed the glomerular membrane, makes up the majority of the urine's protein content. Urine may also contain proteins with lower molecular weights, including globulins. Proteins are almost entirely reabsorbed in the proximal tubule after being filtered at the glomerulus. Therefore, greater glomerular filtration or decreased tubular reabsorption can both lead to proteinuria. Greater protein losses in terms of molecular weight are related to globular proteinuria. Usually, the nephritic condition is accompanied with extraordinarily enormous lassos of protein. Smaller quantities are related to tubular proteinuria (of lower molecular weight protein molecules). Heavy exercise and pregnancy can cause minor protein losses in the urine.

Interpretation

Inflammation, bleeding, or glomerular diseases can all cause proteinuria. Urine that is extremely alkaline or excessively buffered can result in false positive protein results. The most accurate sign of most kidney diseases is proteinuria (nephritic syndrome, nephritic syndrome, tubular disease, urinary tract infections and tumors).

b) Glucose

Glucose is a reducing sugar. In Benedict's reagent, reducing sugar causes cupric ion (Cu^{++}) to change to cuprous ion (Cu^{+}). Depending on the amount of sugar present, cuprous is less soluble and generates cuprous oxide, which yields the colours green, orange, yellow, or red.

Benedict's test

Take 5.0 ml of Benedict's reagent in a test tube; add few drops of the urine. The solution is then boiled vigorously and allowed to cool by it.

Green, orange, yellow or red precipitate means the presence of sugar whereas if sugar is absent, there will not be any colour change.

Colour change	Percentage of sugar
Green	Less than 0.5
Orange	More than 0.5 and less than 1.5
Yellow	1.5
Red	More than 2.0

Clinical significance

Add few drops of the urine to 5.0 ml of Benedict's reagent in a test tube. Then, it vigorously boils the solution and lets it cool.

Precipitate that is green, orange, yellow, or red indicates the presence of sugar, whereas no colour change would occur if sugar were missing.

Interpretation

Since the renal threshold for glucose is greater than 180 mg/dl in most species and 240 mg/dl in cats, glucoseuria is not a typical condition. A proximal renal tubular abnormality or hyperglycemia from diabetes mellitus, an excess of endogenous or exogenous glucocorticoids, or stress can both cause glucosuria (such as primary renal glucosuria).

c) Ketones

In the presence of ammonium hydroxide and ammonium sulphate, nitroprusside interacts with acetoacitic acid to produce permanganate colour.

Rothera's test

Add ammonium sulphate to 5 ml of urine to saturate the urine. Shake after adding 2–3 drops of concentrated ammonium hydroxide and a few drops of freshly made sodium nitroprusside (5%) solution. The appearance of a steadily deepening permanganate tinge is a sign of a positive test.

Clinical significance: When the body is unable to use glucose (as in diabetes) and metabolise fatty acids, ketones flow into the urine. Since this catabolism isn't complete, a lot of acetoacetic acid, acetone, and beta-hydroxybutyric acid are produced (Ketone bodies).

Interpretation

Ketonuria is linked to primary ketosis in ruminants, secondary ketosis in small animals with diabetes mellitus, and occasional prolonged fasting or starvation. If there are reducing substances in the urine, it could result in a false positive reaction.

d) Bile pigment

The yellow compound bilirubin is oxidized by nitric acid into biliverdin (green), bilicynin (blue), bilifusin (brown), choletelin (yellow), etc.

Gmelin test

3.0 ml of concentrated nitric acid should be added to an equal volume of urine in a test tube such that the two liquids don't mix. Note several coloured rings, including green, red, and reddish tallow, at the surface or interface.

Clinical significance and interpretation- Heme degradation results in the formation of bilirubin. It does not end up in the urine. Urine only contains the conjugated form of bilirubin, often known as direct bilirubin. A number of liver conditions including viral hepatitis cause high urine bilirubin levels. When conjugated bilirubin levels surpass the renal threshold due to liver illness or hemolysis, bilirubinuria develops. The main causes of hyperbilirubinuria are bile duct obstruction and moderate to severe hepatocellular damage.

Bile salt

The surface tension of fluids that contain bile salts is reduced.

Sulphur flower test

Pour a little sulphur powder on the surface of 10.0 ml of urine that has been cooled to 17^{0}C or lower in a test tube. If the sulphur settles to the bottom of the urine, bile acid is present.

Clinical significance and interpretation same as bile pigment

e) Occult blood

Haemoglobin acts as a peroxidase enzyme changes Benzidine powder into a coloured compound. H_2O_2 produces a dirty blue or green precipitate that, when left to stand, turns brown.

Benzidine test

Add 2.0 ml of urine & 1.0 ml of hydrogen peroxide to 3.0 ml of a saturated Benzidine in glacial acetic acid solution. A test result is positive when it is blue or green.

Clinical significance and interpretation

Hematuria (hematuria), intravascular hemolysis (hemoglobinuria), or myoglobinuria are all possible causes of a positive reaction. An analysis of the urine sediment under a microscope is necessary to interpret a positive result. Hematuria is a significant indication of glomerulonephritis, stones, tumours, tuberculosis, coagulopathy, infection, vasculitis, schistosomiasis, leptospirosis, and other conditions.

Possible causes for altered values of the following compounds in urine samples

Test	Normal value	Altered values	Possible cause
pH	6.5-7.5	Increased	Microorganisms that produce urease (e.g. Staphylococcus, Proteus)
		Decreased	i) Metabolic acidosis ii) Hypokalaemia iii) Hypochloraemic metabolic alkalosis (uncommon) iv) Renal tubular acidosis
Glucose	Negative or trace	1+ or greater	**Glucose levels over the renal threshold:** i) Diabetes ketoacidosis ii) Starvation iii) Very young animals **Normal serum glucose:** i) Renal tubular disease ii) Primary renal glucosuria

Protein	Negative or trace	2+ or more>1 + in dilute urine	i) Pyruria (infection) ii) Glomerulonephritis or amyloidosis leading to protein-losing nephropathy iii) Haemorrhage iv) Genital tract sections
Ketones	Negative or trace	+1 or greater	i) Diabetic ketoacidosis ii) Starvation iii) Very young animals
Blood	Negative	Positive	i) Haematuria
Haemoglobin	Negative	Positive	i) Intravascular haemolysis (e.g. immune-mediated haemolytic anaemia) ii) Myoglobinuria (due to muscle damage)
Bilirubin	Negative in cats; trace or 1+ in dogs with SG > 1.0252+ in dogs with SG >1.040	Trace/1+ or above in cats	i) Hemolytic anaemia ii) Hepatobiliary disease (especially cats)
Nitrites	Negative	-	Uncontrollable urine retention time in the bladder and frequent false negatives make it unreliable in animals.
Leukocyte esterase	Negative	-	In order to diagnose inflammation in animal urinary tract infections (UTIs), urine sediment must be examined for leucocytes.

Interpretation of urine analysis

C. Microscopic Examination

Method for preparation and analysis

Fresh urine or warmed previously refrigerated urine should be used. A constant volume of urine is placed in a conical centrifuge tube and centrifuge gently (1,000 rpm for 5 minutes) to prevent cast destruction. The high speed may also damage cells and destroy casts. The supernatant is decanted. A few drops of liquid will remain in the tube. A drop of sediment is placed on a clean glass slide and a cover slip is placed over it to avoid air bubbles. The slide is placed on microscope stage and the whole area is scanned on low power (10X objective). The presence of crystal is reported as 1+, 2+. 3+. or light, moderate, heavy. Identification of crystal type should be attempted. The number of erythrocytes, leucocytes and epithelial cells, casts, crystals and bacteria seen per high power field are counted and recorded.

Unless there are really huge numbers present, it is best to count in 5–10 distinct fields and then average the results. Other components, such as sperm, mucus stands, yeast, fungus, nematode eggs, and fat droplets, have been described. The 100X oil emersion objective can be used to better identify cell types or to distinguish bacteria from particles. ? Fine focusing and adjusting the condenser typically allow one to discriminate between fat and air bubbles. At 100X power, motile bacteria may typically be differentiated from Brownian motion of particles.

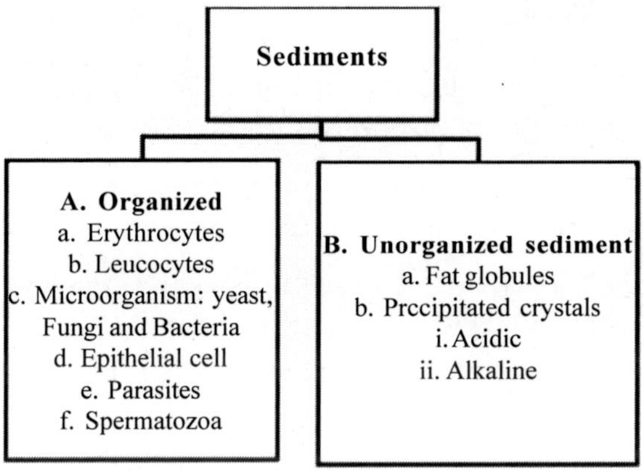

Classification of sediments

Erythrocytes

Erythrocytes are non-uniform in sized and spherical in shape, resembling shadow cells with a faint ring of colour. They are smaller than leucocytes. The erythrocytes balloon if the urine has a low specific gravity and low concentration. These have a distorted look because to their crenated periphery. Erythrocytes seen in urine are a sign of genitourinary system haemorrhage. The urethra is the source of haemorrhage if the blood appears as animals/human start to urinate. The last portion of the urine in a bladder haemorrhage is combined with blood, whereas the last portion of the urine in a kidney haemorrhage is mixed with urine and blood. Cathodization, bladder puncture, and bladder manipulation can all result in haemorrhage.

Leucocytes

WBC's are slightly larger than RBC and have grainy cytoplasm. Normal urine should contain <5 WBC/ field at 400X magnification. Increase WBC (pyuria) can occur due to inflammation, infection, trauma or Neoplasia. Catherization or collection of voided urine may introduce a few WBC from the urogenital tract. Ten or more WBC/ mm^3 of urine indicate urinary tract infection.

Epithelial cells

The cells are often visible in urine, despite being few. In cases of cystitis or other inflammatory conditions of the urinary tract, the number of epithelial cells rises. Urine contains squamous epithelial cells from the urethra, bladder, and vagina. These sediment cells are the biggest ones and feature little rounded nuclei. Leucocytes are larger than renal tubule epithelial cells, which are smaller, spherical or polyhedral in shape.

Microorganism

Any infectious disease of the urinary tract involves the presence of microorganisms. Urine may contain bacteria, yeast, fungus, or protozoa as the organisms.

1. **Bacteria:** Can be found in pyelonephritis and cystitis, and can be recognised by Gram's staining.
2. **Yeast**: these are colourless, round to avoid bodies with double refractile walls and these are usually contaminants.
3. **Fungi**: Hyphae on fungi are distinctively segmented. Colored fungus are meaningless.

Parasites

The urine sediment of the following parasites may include their ova.

- Swine kidney worm- *Stephanurus dentatus*
- Dog and mink giant kidney worms- *Dioctophyma renale*
- Dog, cat, and fox bladder worms - *Capillaria plica*
- Due to urine contamination of faeces, *Dirofilaria immitis*- microfilaria may be present in the urine (rarely) and several parasitic eggs. Trichomonads and Giardia are genital tract contaminants; protozoa, which are uncommon in urine, are faecal contaminants.

Spermatozoa

Easily recognizable by their shape and common in the urine of male dogs (less common in other species).

Cylindruria (Casts)

Casts are long, cylindric structures that can contain cells and are created when renal tubules and mucoprotein congeal. Mucoprotein makes up hyaline casts, which have parallel sides and rounded ends. They can happen when you have a fever, exercise, or renal disease. Entrapment of shed tubular epithelial cells in the mucoprotein results in epithelial cellular casts, which can be seen in patients with renal impairment. It is believed that granular casts are degraded epithelial cellular casts. Typically, they have shattered ends and sharp borders. Erythrocyte and WBC casts are examples of further cellular casts. Renal haemorrhage is the cause of erythrocyte cast formation.

As with pyelonephritis, renal inflammation causes WBC casts. Although they are uncommon, fatty casts can be seen in people with lipid metabolic problems like diabetes mellitus. The presence of a few hyaline or granular casts is normal. The appearance of cellular casts or other casts in significant quantities, however, denotes renal injury and may be one of the initial laboratory abnormalities associated with renal epithelial cell damage caused by toxic agents (e.g. gentamicin, amphotericin B).

Hyaline casts: normal finding.

WBC casts: acute pyelonephritis

RBC casts: nephritic syndrome or necrotizing glomerulopathy

Epithelial cell casts: tubulointestinal disease

Fatty casts (i.e. fat within tubular epithelium): nephritic syndrome

Waxy and broad casts: renal disease

Crystals

The pH, solubility, and concentration of the crystalloid and colloidal depend on whether there are crystals in the urine. These are not clinically significant when present. Amorphous urates, uric acid, and less frequently calcium oxalate and hippuric acids, may be present in normal acidic urine. Triple and amorphous phosphate, calcium carbonate (particularly in horse urine), and infrequently ammonium urate crystals may be seen in alkaline urine. Except when urolithiasis is observed because of a change in protein metabolism and may result in cystine calculi, aberrant crystals in urine are of little consequence.

Fat

These appear as round and highly refractile bodies of varying sizes. Sudan III stain causes these to turn orange to crimson. They typically come from unrelated sources like a greasy container or a lubricated catheter. Most cats experience lipuria, or the presence of fat in the urine, on a regular basis. This condition can result from renal tubule fatty transformation, lymphatic rupture, obesity, diabetes mellitus, hypothyroidism, and animals that consume a high-fat diet.

Dipsticks: Today, the urine's colour and smell (if any) are noted, and urine chemistries are carried out using reagent strips with coloured pads (such as "Multistix" or "Chemstrip").

Utilizing these is simple. Before dipping the stick, stir the urine. Don't touch the pads. Don't let the strip sit in the urine for too long. Don't let the dye run.

Department of Veterinary Clinical Complex

Format of Urine Test

Urine analysis ....

Animal species: ....

Owner name: .... Gender: ....

Breed: .... Age: ....

Referred by: .... Date: ....

Test Result: ....

Physical	Test	Observation	Interpretation
	pH	....	....
	Specific gravity	....	....
	Turbidity	....	....
	Casts	....	....
	Crystals	....	....
Chemical	**Glucose**	....	....
	Fehling's test	....	....
	Benedict's test	....	....
	Ketone bodies	....	....
	Rothera's test	....	....
	Proteins	....	....
	Heat coagulationTest	....	....
	Heller's test	....	....
	Bilirubin	....	....
	Gmelin test	....	....
	Fouchet's test	....	....
	Bile salts	....	....
	Hay's test	....	....
	Blood	....	....
	Benzidine test	....	....
	Urobilinogen	....	....
	i.Ehrlich's test	....	....
Microscopic	Infectious organism	....	....
	Blood cells	....	....
	Epithelial cells	....	....
	Miscellaneous	....	....

Comment on the case: ....

....

....

Signature of Incharge

Questions

1. What are the different physical properties for urine analysis?
2. Define Rothera's test?
3. Define Heller's ring test?
4. Write name of few parasites eggs which can be seen in urine sediments?
5. Write importance of microscopic examination of urine?

9

Clinical Hematology in Veterinary Practice

Rajesh Kumar Verma

Collections of blood

To collect blood for different haematological analyses, an animal's vein are punctured with a syringe and needle.

Requirements

- Hypodermic needle
- Syringe
- Collection vials or tubes containing anticoagulants.

Procedure

- The place of blood collection should always be cleaned with alcohol and hairs trimmed.
- Press on the vein to raise it.
- Free-flowing blood can be collected directly into the vial containing anticoagulant after the needle is inserted into the vein.
- 5 ml of blood from large animals and 2.0 ml of blood from small animals like dogs and cats are sufficient for normal haematological investigations.
- Rotational motions in the vials are used to mix the blood.

Precaution

- Always take the recommended dosage of an anticoagulant. A surplus of it will lead to PCV errors and cellular morphological deformation.
- Always use a dry, sterilized needle and syringe.
- Avoid forcefully shaking the blood for concern that foam would form, rupture the red blood cells, and allow adequate space for mixing in vial.
- Fresh blood should be used to make blood smears, ideally within 15 minutes of blood collection.

Site of blood collection

S. No.	Animals	Sites
1.	Cattle and buffaloes	Jugular vein, ear vein
2.	Horses	Jugular vein
3.	Camel	Jugular vein
4.	Sheep	Jugular vein
5.	Goat	Jugular vein
6.	Pig	Ear vein, anterior vena cave,
7.	Dog	Cephalic vein, recurrent tarsal vein
8.	Poultry	Wing vein, heart

Haematological tests for convenience can be categorized as follows

A.	Erythrocyte related tests	Haemoglobin estimationPacked cell volumeTotal erythrocyte count
B.	Leukocyte related tests	Total leukocyte countDifferential leukocyte count
C.	General/ non specific	Erythrocyte sedimentation rate

Haemoglobin Estimation

The erythrocyte contains 400 billion haemoglobin molecules, accounting for 95% of its dry weight. Haeme and globin combine to form the conjugated protein known as haemoglobin.

There are four ways to estimate haemoglobin. For clinical objectives, two procedures are usually applied. Both are colorimetric.

1. **Direct method:** Color standard is used to compare the depth of colour. This involves applying a drop of blood to filter paper, which is then compared to a standard that has been coloured on lithographs.
    - Tallquist haemoglobin scale
    - Dare haemoglobinometer
2. **Oxyhaemoglobin method**: Oxyhaemoglobin is not produced from methaemoglobin or carboxyhemoglobin. Lower values are obtained when functional haemoglobin is measured.
3. **Cyanmethaemoglobin method:** Best method measures almost all types of circulating haemoglobin.
4. Sahli's acid haematin method:

Principle: The dilute hydrochloric acid (N/ 10 HCl), which is added, converts the haemoglobin into acid haematin. The resultant brownish yellow colour is matched with the standard comparator or colorimeter.

Requirements

- Sahli's haemoglobinometer, it consists of following-
- Comparator of brownish/ amber coloured
- Sahli's haemoglobinometer glass tube with marking of gram percent/ percentage of haemoglobin.
- Sahli's pipette having marking of 20mm
- N (N/10) HCl
- Distill water
- Glass stirrer

Procedure

- Rotation of the specimen tube while the blood and anticoagulants are mixed
- Fill the haemoglobin approximated tube with N/ 10 HCl to the mark 10 on the percentage side or the mark 2 g percent on the other side.
- Fill the pipette with exactly 20 μl of blood.
- Wipe the pipette's tip.
- Insert the pipette into the tube containing the N/10 HCl. Suck the contents into the pipette and repeatedly discharge them into the HCl.
- Stir the mixture in a circular motion with a stirrer and let it stand for 5–10 minutes.
- Drop by drop, while stirring; dilute the mixture with distilled water until the colour is identical with the standard.
- Take note of the reading from Sahli's tube and the Hb concentration (in grammes per 100 millilitres of blood).

Precaution

- Mix the blood samples by rotation.
- Remove any extra blood by wiping the pipette's outer surface.
- Give sufficient time for the chemical reaction to complete.

Source of Error

- Using a pipette that has been damaged.
- Taking an insufficient amount of blood.
- Excessive acid consumption.
- Not waiting long enough for the colour to develop as recommended.

Packed Cell Volume (PCV) Estimation/ Haematocrit

Haematocrit is the percentage of total volume occupied by packed erythrocytes when a known given volume of blood is centrifuged for a constant period of time at a constant period.

Methods of estimation

Two methods:

- Macrohaematocrit or Wintrobe tube
- Microhaematocrit method

1. Macrohaematocrit or Wintrobe tube methods

Requirements

- Anticoagulant added blood sample
- Wintrobe tube- it is a test tube having 3 mm bore. It is calibrated doubly with 10 cm scale having millimeter divisions. The scale on the right side is read from bottom to top (0 to 10) for PCV and left in the reverse (10 to 0) for ESR. The tube can hold 1 ml of blood. The percentage volume of each blood compartment is determined by reading directly on the scale. The time and speed of centrifugation are important.
- Dry syringe with 5-6 inches blunt needle (16-18 gauges).
- Centrifuge machine.

Procedure

- Haematocrit is the percentage of total volume occupied by packed erythrocytes when a known volume of blood is centrifuged for a constant period of time at a constant period.
- Stir the blood sample thoroughly in a circular motion to ensure that the cells are suspended uniformly.
- Draw blood using a Pasteur pipette or a syringe with a 6" aspirator needle that has a blunt end.
- Insert the Pasteur pipette or needle into the tube's bottom.
- As the tube fills exactly to the "0" point, slowly expel the blood while raising the pipette.
- When filling, care must be taken to ensure that the needle's tip (opening) is always below the blood column.
- Prevent air bubbles.

- For the blood of dogs and horses, place the tube in a centrifuge and rotate at 3000 rpm for 30 minutes; for the blood of cattle, sheep, goats, and pigs, rotate for 60 minutes.
- Read the PCV after removing the tube.
- The erythrocyte will be packed at the bottom and leukocytes and platelets in between (Buffy coat) and the plasma at the top

$$PCV = \frac{\text{Height of RBC column in mm X100 \%}}{\text{Total height of column in mm}}$$

Error

2.25 to 8.5 percent. Sources of errors are-

- Insufficient time and centrifugation
- Not utilizing the proper dosage of an anticoagulant

Advantages of Macrohaematocrit

- Understanding the nature of plasma
- No expensive machinery is required.
- An approximate estimate of the leukocyte count can be made.

Disadvantages

- More blood is needed.
- Centrifugation takes more time.
- PCV is not accurate since the amount of trapped plasma is more.

Microhaematocrit method

Procedure

- Gently rotate the blood that contains anticoagulant.
- Place the capillary tube's one end on the blood's surface.
- Blood enters the tube by rising due to capillary action. Remove the tube when it is two-thirds full & seal the end with plasticine, paraffin, or a flame.
- Insert the capillary tube into the groove of the unique centrifuge with the sealed end facing outward.
- Securely fasten the centrifuge's cover, and then spin it for two minutes (12000G).
- A reader scale that comes with the device is used to read the PCV.

Microcapillary tubes with coated or uncoated oxalates are available in two sizes of 7.5 cm X 1.0 mm and 3.2 cm X 0.08 mm.

Even by Microhaematocrit method the blood of sheep and goats require longer centrifugation time (10-12 min). For others 5 min is sufficient.

Advantages of Microhaematocrit

- One of the benefits of microhaematocrit is that very little blood is needed.
- Centrifugation must be completed in less time.
- The PCV is more precise since there is almost no trapped plasma in the space between the erythrocytes.

Disadvantages

- ESR cannot be estimated.
- Buffy's coat is too thin and difficult to read, and the plasma colour is unnoticeable.
- An expensive, specialized centrifuge is required.

Total Erythrocyte Count Estimation

Methods

- Haemocytometer method- Cheap and the best.
- Electronic counting method- High cost.

Haemocytometer Method

Principle

Accurate dilution of a measured quality of blood with a fluid which is isotonic with the blood and count erythrocyte in counting chamber.

Requirement

- Anticoagulant-treated blood samples.
- Thoma pipette with a red bead in the bulb for dilution. Graduated from 0.5-101.
- Diluting fluids

Diluting fluids

A. Normal saline

B. Hayem's solution

Mercuric chloride	0.5 mg
Sodium chloride	1.5 mg
Sodium sulphate	5.0 mg
Distilled water	200 ml

There may be agglutination in blood when the solution becomes more than 2-3 weeks old.

C. Grower's solution

Sodium sulphate anhydrous	12.5g
Glacial acetic acid	33.3 ml
Distilled water	200ml

Counting not good as agglutination is common.

Procedure

- Mix the blood sample with anticoagulant by rotation.
- Use an RBC diluting pipette to draw blood up to the 0.5 mark. Wipe away any extra blood, and if the line is crossed, remove the rubber tubing and mix the contents for two to three minutes while holding the pipette horizontally between the thumb and middle finger.
- Drain the pipette at least1/3 part of the way and clean the tip (purpose is to remove fluid in capillary portion of the pipette which has not mixed with blood).
- Fill the hemocytometer with blood by placing the pipette tip between the counting chambers, and the cover glass.
- Allow the cells about 3 minutes to set, but keep them from evaporating.
- Count cells in Central Square of the 9 large squares. Under high power, count erythrocyte in 5 of the 25 small squares in the central area following principle of double ruling or triple ruling.
- Any variation of more than 10% in one of the five centre squares indicates unequal distribution and necessitates the haemocytometer being recharged.

Calculation of erythrocytes/mm^3

= Cells counted x (10 (0.1 mm depth) x 5 (1/5 of sq. mm) x 200 (1: 200 dilution)

= Sum of cells in 5 small squares x 10,000

Erythrocytic Sedimentation Rate Estimation

The distance by which the erythrocytes fall during a given period of time is measured in millimeter (mm) and is known as ESR.

Principle

A tube containing blood to which an anticoagulant has been added is place in vertical position; erythrocytes sink because they are heavier than the plasma in which they are suspended. The distance that erythrocytes fall during a given period of time is measured.

Methods

A. Wintrobe tube method

B. Westergren method

A. Wintrobe tube method

Requirement

- Anticoagulant added blood sample.
- Dry syringe with 4-6 inch long needle (16-18 gauze).
- Wintrobe tube with steel rack

Procedure

- The Wintrobe tube is filled to the 0 mark on the left side.
- The tube is set in the appropriate rack vertically.
- For particular animal species, the upper level of sedimentation, or erythrocytes, is measured in mm on the left scale at time intervals as specified below:

Animals	Time period
Buffalo/ Horse	10, 20 or 30 min
Cattle	8 or 24 hrs
Sheep and Goat	24 hrs
Dog, cat	1 hrs

The results are expressed as fall of R.B.C's in mm/hr.

B. Westergren method

Requirement

- Blood sample containing anticoagulant
- Westergren tube with stand

Procedure

- Fill up the western tube (Total length of 300 mm, 2 mm diameter, a capacity of 1 ml and graduation from 0-200 at 1 mm intervals) up to the 0 mark by aspiration.
- The tube is fixed in upright position in a special rack with a soft rubber cushion at the bottom so that tube is sealed when inserted.
- Record the fall of erythrocytes in mm at various intervals as mentioned in Wintrobe tube method.

Sources of error and precautions

- The temperature of refrigerated samples should be maintained because it affects the ESR and vice versa.
- The Wintrobe tube should be perfectly perpendicular.
- Air bubble trapping should be avoided because it affects rate.
- The tube needs to be set up in a space free from disturbance or vibrations.
- The tube needs to be dry and clean.
- It is not recommended to haemolyze the blood sample.

Total leukocyte count determination

The number of leukocytes in peripheral blood in a given unit of blood is total leukocyte count.

Haemocytometer methods

Requirements

- Anticoagulant added sample.
- Haemocytometer with special cover glass
- Pipette with a white bead in the bulb for dilution. Graduated from 0.5-11.
- WBC diluting fluid Microscope

Turk's Fluids

Glacial acetic acid	2 ml
Gentian violet (1% aqueous)	1 ml
Distilled water	100 ml

Filter before use.

Procedure

- Mix the blood sample by rotation.
- Take the blood in the WBC dilution pipette up to the 0.5 mark (after connecting with rubber tubing) and wipe the blood from the outside.
- Draw diluting liquid up to the 11-point mark above the bulb.
- Remove the rubber tubing and mix the contents while holding the pipette horizontally for two to three minutes.
- Before filling the counting chamber, throw away the first few of drops (about a third of the pipette).
- Load the haemocytometer by touching the tip of pipette in space between edge and cover glass.
- Leave leukocytes two minutes to settle and for the lysis of erythrocytes.
- Count the cells under low power magnification (x 10) in four corner large squares (each is divided in 16 small squares) by following the exclusion principle of cells counting along the line as discussed in TEC.

Calculation

TLC/ mm^3= cell counted x 20 (1: 20 dilution) x10 (0.1 depth)/ 4 (No. of sq. mm. counted) =Sum of WBCs in squares x 50.

Differential Leukocyte Count Determination

The differential count can be made by counting 100 cells in well stained blood smear and classifying different cells the examination of well stained blood smear by a knowledgeable observer can provide more valuable information than any other single laboratory test.

There are two methods for preparing blood smear

1. Coverslip method-Distribution of cells is best but difficult to handle & clean.
2. Slide method- Slide blood smear can easily be made and give adequate results and routinely followed. The method is described in detail:

Requirements

Fresh blood/sample collected in anticoagulant preferably with EDTA.

- Clean, dry slides with smooth edges.
- Strains- Giemsa, Leishman
- Methanol/ ethyl alcohol/formaldehyde.
- Applicator stick/ capillary tube.
- Mechanical cell counter.

Characteristic of a good blood smear

- It should be feathery and thin at one end and thick at the other.
- At least 2 mm should separate the film's edge from the edge of the slide.
- The smear must to seem smooth and be devoid of any gaps.
- Presences of holes indicate grease on slide/ spreader. There should not be any jerk in it.
- It should cover two thirds of the slide.
- It should have a tongue-like form.

Procedure

- Mix the blood sample by rotation
- Take blood on dry grease free smooth edged slide near blood drop to 2/3rd of slide, the spreader is gently pushed to draw blood smear.
- By waving in the air and avoiding blowing, the stain is dried.
- For three minutes, fix the smear with methanol (not necessary when using the Wright & Leishman or Ramenowsky strain).

Giemsa staining

- If the smear is not already set and dried, fix it in methanol for 3 minutes.
- Flood the slide placed over glass bars/ use coplin jar (for using diluted Giemsa stain 1: 10) with distilled water/ buffered water (pH 6.8).
- Give the smear 30 minutes to stain. Giemsa can be used diluted for a staining process that takes about 10 to 15 minutes.
- Wash with distill water, dry and examine under microscope.

Leishman's stain

Procedure for staining

- Apply Leishman's stain over the blood stain for 1-3 minutes.
- Add double quantity of buffer of pH 6.6 and mix by blowing air. When properly mixed a greenish metallic sheen will form. The buffer makes the stain to penetrate into cells.
- Held it for 10 minutes.
- After 10 minutes, wash with a stream of tap water.
- Immediately wipe and dry the bottom of the slide.
- Set the films in upright position on a dryer rack then examine under microscope (100X).

Defects in staining of slides

No.	Defect	Cause
1.	Entire blood smear is too blue, granules of eosinophils overstained and larger.	Too alkaline buffered water/ wash water/ stain-Exercise thick smear
		Alkaline residue on slide
		Insufficient washing
		Prolonged stained before diluting with buffered water.
2.	Leukocyte nuclei pale blue R.B.C. and eosinophilic granules unusually red.	Too acidic buffered water/ wash/ stain
		Acidic residue on slide.
3.	Entire smear has pale stain	Old/ Weak stain
		Exercise washing
		Using warm/ hot water for washing slide
4.	Variation in staining on different areas of smear	Buffered water unevenly applied or not thoroughly mixed
		Acid/ alkaline residue on slide
		Water not properly drained from slide after washing.
5.	Precipitated stain	Lack of thorough washing
		Precipitate in Wright's stain (not properly filtered)
		Evaporation of alcoholic stain due to excessive staining time.
		Tilting of slide to one and side and stain runs down.

The demonstration of haemoprotozoan can be done along with DLC. Some important tips for identification include

Trypanosomes: The demonstration of flagellates in the thin or thick blood films or by biological test by inoculation in laboratory animals is used for diagnosis.

Anaplasma: the demonstration of characteristic organisms in erythrocytes is used for diagnosis.

Babesia: the demonstration of characteristic piroplasmic stages in the erythrocytes from peripheral blood film is used for diagnosis.

Theileria: the demonstration of Koch's blue bodies in the lymphocytes and monocytes of the lymph node smear or peripheral blood film is pathognomonic of disease.

Interpretation of HB, PCV and TEC

A. Polycythemia- (Increased TEC with corresponding increase in Hb and PCV)

   i) **Relative:** (More erythrocytes per unit of blood volume, but no more production): Dehydration, water restriction, diarrheal vomiting, excessive perspiration, shift of bodily fluids to intestinal tissue, shock, and burns are some of the symptoms.

   ii) **Absolute:** (Increased number of erythrocytes because of increased production)

      a) **Primary:** Polycythemia vera (dog, cat, cattle and man- unknown cause), Familial Polycythemia (man and jersey calves- Hereditary)

      b) **Secondary:** Increased RBC production stimulation, Chronic lung and heart illness, hypoxia, high altitude, methaemoglobinemia, sulphhaemoglobinemia, biological, newborn, Cobalt poisoning, local hypoxia, increased erythropoietin production, renal cyst and hydronephrosis.

B. **Oligocythermia (Anaemia):** (Decreased below normal TEC, Hb and PCV).

Types

I. **Microcytic hypochromic (MCV decreased):** Chronic haemorrhages, parasites that feed on blood, & a lack of iron, copper, pyridoxine, & riboflavin.

II. **Microcytic normochromic (MCV decreased):** Radiation injury, Bracken fern toxicity, and Soyabean poisoning (Trichloroethylene extracted).

III. **Macrocytic hyperchromatic (MCV increased):** Transitory following acute haemorrhage, Sweet clover poisoning, Bacillary Haemoglobinuria, Leptospirosis, Postparturient Haemoglobinuria, Anaplasmosis, Piroplasmosis, Haemobartnellosis.

IV. **Macrocytic normochromic (MCV increased):** Vit B12 deficiency, Folic acid increased bone marrow activity (transitory following acute haemorrhages).

V. **Normocytic normochromic (MCHC normal):** Anaemia of decreased production, Aplastic anaemia, Inherited enzyme deficiency, acute haemorrhage, Autoimmune disease of new borns, Incompatible blood transfusion.

VI. **Normocytic hypochromic (MCHC decreased):** Stomach worm infection excluding Haemonchus, Leukemia, Hypoplastic anaemias.

VII. **Hyperchromic (normocytic/ Macrocytic/ Microcytic):** No condition as RBCs can't be supersaturated.

Interpretation of Erythrocytic Sedimentation Rate

It is a general test to assess the severity of a disease process within the body.

1. The probability of illness cannot be ruled out with a normal ESR.
2. It is unsuccessful in horses and buffalo and more effective in dogs, cats, and pigs (very rapid because there is an intense rouleax formation). Cattle, sheep, and goats do not exhibit rouleax formation (clumping of RBCs), which is only mildly visible in cats, pigs, and dogs.

Increased ESR

A. General conditions

Acute generalized infections, acute localized infections of serosal membranes peritonitis and pericarditis, suppurative conditions, malignant neoplasms, Hyperadrenocorticism, pregnancy (increased fibrinogen), hypothyroidism, tissue injury/ destruction including surgery.

B. Specific conditions

Dog: Canine distemper, Leptospirosis, Pregnancy, Pyometra, Neoplasms, Chronic intestinal nephritis, Infectious canine hepatitis, Endocarditis, myocarditis, Hypothyroidism, Hyperadrenocorticism, Filariasis, Pneumonia, pleuritis Trypanosomiasis, Bone fracture

Horse: Equine infectious anaemia, Strongyloides infection

Cattle: Normal in pregnancy

Decreased ESR

Dog: Liver disease (low plasma protein), Poor nutrition More immature RBCs

Horse: Hyperglobilinemias

Interpretation of TLC and DLC

Total leukocyte count varies in certain physiological conditions which include: Age of animal, breed of species of animal, excitement and muscular activity, stage of pregnancy, stage of estrus and digestion. These factors should be considered while interpreting results.

Leucopenia

(Decrease in absolute count of leukocytes)

- Viral diseases: Canine distemper, feline panleukopenia, infectious canine hepatitis, hog cholera, Rinder pest, Swine influenza, malignant catarrhal fever.
- Bacterial infection in early age.
- localized severe infections.
- Toxoplasmosis
- Sequestration of Europhiles in shock
- Bone marrow abnormalities
- Chemicals
- Drugs (Chloramphenicol, aspirin)

Neutropenia

(Decrease in absolute count of neutrophils)

- Overwhelming bacterial/ viral infections
- Shock
- Bone marrow depression
- Deficiency of Vit. B_{12} and folic acid

Eosinopenia

(Decreased in absolute count of eosinophils)

- Stress
- Intoxications
- Trauma
- Hyperadrenocorticism

Lymphopenia

(Decrease in absolute count of lymphocytes)

- Viral diseases: Hog cholera, Infectious canine hepatitis, Canine distemper, Bovine viral diarrhea.
- Hyper adrenocorticism
- Radiation
- Immune suppressive drugs
- Chronic enteric disease

Leukocytosis

(Increase in absolute count of leukocytes)

- Physiological: Strenuous exercise, convulsion, excitement, fear, digestion and pregnancy.
- Pathological: Localized/ generalized infections) Staphylococci, Streptococci, Corynebacterium.
- Acute blood loss, haemorrhage, hetrolysis.
- Intoxications: Uremia, acidosis, diabetes, chemicals (Pb, Hg) foreign protein reaction and snake/ insect venom
- Tissue necrosis: Infraction, burn, gangrene, neoplasm
- Adrenal corticoids
- Trauma particularly following surgery

Neutrophilia

(Increase in absolute count of Europhiles)

- Inflammation: Bacterial, rickettsial, mycotic and parasitic
- Trauma
- Neoplasia
- Intoxictaion
- Surgical procedures
- Hyperadrenocorticism
- Metabolic and endocrine disorders
- Localized suppurative
- Shift to left: Increase in immature neutrophils (above 6% of TLC) poor prognosis.
- Shift to right: Increase in number of mature neutrophils (Horse shoe or multiplied nucleus) good prognosis.
- Schilling index to express the increase in mature/ immature neutrophils.

Lymphocytosis

(Increase in absolute count of lymphocytes)

- Physiological in calves and kittens
- Chronic infections
- After vaccination
- Autoimmune disease
- Lymphocytic leukemia
- Hypoadrenocortism
- Relative lymphocytes along with leucopenia and Neutropenia
- Lymphadenitis/ lymphangitis

Eosinophilia

(Increase in absolute count of eosinophils)

- Parasitism: Filariasis, Hookworm, lungworm, Trichinosis, Fascioliasis, Strongylosis, Spirocerosis
- Allergic: Allergic bronchitis, hay fever, skin allergies, anaphylactic reaction
- Adrenocortical insufficiency
- Diseases of organs rich in mast cells i.e. skin, lung GIT and female genital tract (during estrus)
- Eosinophilic myositis
- Protozoa: Babesiosis, theileriasis
- Chronic condition of skin (subcutaneous), lung, GIT uterus scrotum and serosal lining.

Monocytosis

(Increase in absolute count of monocytes)

- Corticoids in dogs and cattle
- Recovery/ late phase of acute disease
- All chronic supportive diseases
- Granulomatous conditions- Tuberculosis, Brucellosis, Mycotic (Systemic) infections
- Disease with tissue debris: hemorrhages exudates in cavities, Pyometra, retained placenta

- Monocytic leukemia in canine
- Stress

Basophilia

(Increase in absolute count of basophils)

- Associated with Eosinophilia e.g. heart worms, chronic respiratory disease
- Basophilic leukemia
- Hypothyroidism
- Hyperadrenocorticism in dogs.

Normal Haemogram of different animals and poultry

Species	Hemoglobin (gm/dl)	Packed cell volume (%)	Total erythrocyte count (x 10^6/	ESR value (mm/ hr)
Cattle	8-14(11)	26-42(34)	5-8(7)	2.25-4/ 24 hrs
Buffalo	10.8-13.3	30-41	5.8-6.2	55-60/hr
Goat	8-14(11)	20-38 (28)	8-17 (13)	2-2.5/ 24 hrs
Sheep	8-16(12)	24-45 (35)	8-15 (12)	3-8.5/ 24 hrs
Horse	11-18 (15)	32-52 (42)	7-13 (9)	61-63/hr
Pig	10-16 (13)	32-50 (45)	5-8 (6.5)	5.5-11/24 hrs
Cat	8-15 (12)	24-45 (37)	6-9 (6.8)	15.4/hr
Dog	12-18 (15)	37-54(42)	7-13 (9)	5-25/hr
Camel	11.9	30.08	6.1-7.3(7.26)	....
Elephant	12-15.5(13-14)	38.20	6.1-7.3	....
Guinea pig	11-17 (14)	33-45 (40)	4-7 (6)	....
Rabbit	8-15 (12)	30-50 (40)	4-7 (6)	....
Rat	11-18 (15)	35-45 (45)	7-10 (9)	....
Fowl	8.83-11.3	27-42	2.18-4.12	1.5/hr

Normal Haemogram of domestic animal, poultry and man

Species	MCV (μ^3)	MHC (μμg)	MCHC (%)	TLC ($x10^3$)	N(%)	L (%))	M (%))	E(%)	B (%)
Cattle	40-60 (52)	11-17 (14)	30-36 (33)	4-12 (5.6)	15-45	48-75	2-7	2-15	0-2
Buffalo	-	-	-	10.61	43-45	45-48	-	3-4	-
Goat	15-30 (23)	10-12.6	35-42 (38)	6-16 (12)	30-48	50-70	1-4	3-8	0-2
Sheep	23-48 (33)	9-12 (10.7)	31-38(33)	4-12 (5.6)	10-50	40-75	1-5	1-8	0-3
Horse	34-58(46)	12-18(15)	31-37(35)	7-14(8.8)	30-65	25-70	1-8	1-10	0-3
Pig	50-68(63)	17-23(20)	30-34(32)	11-22(16)	28-47	39-60	2-10	1-11	0-2
Cat	19-55(45)	13-17(15)	30-36(33)	8-25(13.8)	35-75	22-55	1-4	2-10	rare
Dog	60-77(70)	19-25(23)	32-36(43)	5.6-19(19.7)	60-75	12-30	3-9	2-10	rare
Camel	55	21-49	25-39	20.07	38.7	46	5-7	9.5	1
Elephant	143-146(145)	41-44	29-31	6.4-14(10.16)	22-50(36.5)	40-60(51.7)	1.7-5(2)	6-15(9)	0-3.2
Guinea pig	83	25	34	7-14(10)	30-50(42)	35-55(45)	10-20	2-15(5)	0-2(0.5)
Rabbit	68.0	7-24	0-35	6-12	17-52	42-80	5-8	0-3	0-5
Rat	57-65	18-22	31.7-35	5-23(14)	8-40(20)	50-80(60)	2-7(5)	0-4(2)	0-2(1)
Fowl	127	37	29	20-35(33.3)	29.5-37.3	48.9-58.4	9.7-10.2	1.7	0.7-2

Questions

1. What is dilution factor for TLC count?
2. Name one condition in which there is Leukocytosis?
3. How many tertiary squares are taken to count TEC?
4. Name one condition in which there is erythrocytosis?
5. Why fixation is not necessary while staining the blood smear with Leishman's stain?
6. Name two stains which can be used for staining blood smears for screening blood protozoan?
7. Name few intracellular and extra cellular blood protozoans?
8. Name one disease of cattle in which ESR is significantly increased?
9. Draw the diagram of various leukocytes in the blood smear?

Proforma for Blood Examination

S. No.: .... **Date: ....**

Owner name: .... Case no.: ....
Animal Species: .... Breed: ....
Sex: .... Age: ....
Clinician: ....
Test required Anticoagulant used: ....
Time of collection Time of receiving: ....
Total Leucocyte Count / mm^3: ....
Differential Leucocyte Count: ....
Neutrophils: .... % ....
Lymphocyte: .... % ....
Eosinophils: .... % ....
Basophils: .... % ....
Monocytes: .... % ....
Total erythrocyte count: .... / mm^3 ....
Haemoglobin: .... Gm% ....
E.S.R.:.. mm fall in Ist hour...
Total platelets: .... / mm^3..
Absolute Eosinophil:.......................... / mm^3..
PCV (%): ....
MCV: .... fl ....
MCH: .... Picograms (pg) per cell ....
MCHC: .... g/dl ....
Haemoprotozoan: ....
Remarks: ....

Time: .... **Date:...**

Signature

10

Parasitic Diseases Laboratory Evaluation and Diagnosis of Samples

Rajesh Kumar Verma

Purpose of study

An essential component of the diagnostic process in the evaluation of the disease process is the laboratory diagnosis of any parasitic infection. Sometimes, this confirms the presumptive clinical diagnosis, and other times, it provides evidence that the clinician may have ignored. A sufficient specimen must be used for the examination to achieve a satisfactory diagnosis. Internal parasite testing needs to be done often. Regular inspection typically enables early parasitism identification, preventing gross infection. The majority of the parasites can be accurately identified by doing a detailed examination of the faeces.

Faecal sample collection and delivery for parasite identification

The faecal sample is collected directly from the animal. When handling large animals, one should put on gloves, wet their hands, and collect the faeces from the rectum. If there are no faeces in the rectum, massage the mucosa with the finger, and the animal will defecate in a short period of time. Put 5–10 g of faeces in a dry, transparent glass container. In order to collect faeces for cultural analysis, glass vials should be sanitised. The faeces of small animals like calves, sheep, goats, and dogs are collected using the index finger. The cloacal swabs from poultry are collected for analysis. If a sample of freshly defecated faeces is being taken, the middle portion should be taken and should be free of mud, dirt, and foreign objects.

Storage

The faeces should always be examined as soon as possible after collection. The faeces should be kept in a refrigerator at 40 degrees Celsius, though, if examination-related deterioration is expected. It must be brought from a distant location to the lab, appropriately sealed, and marked. Additionally, 10% formalin might be administered to the faeces as a preservative for parasite examination. Without adding any preservative, the faeces sample taken for lungworm larval investigation should be put into sealed containers.

Examination of faeces

1. **Gross examination:** The faecal sample is kept in clean, dry petridishes for gross examination. With the help of spatula or clean glass rod, it should be spread properly and examined for its colour, consistency, odour and presence of blood, parasite, segments of parasite or any other foreign material.
2. **Microscopic examination:** Routinely the microscopic examination of faeces is performed by following methods: 1. Direct examination and 2. Concentration methods consisting of sedimentation and flotation techniques.

A. Direct wet mount

1. A small quantity of faeces about the size of a pin's head is placed on a slide.
2. Two or three drops of water are added.
3. The faeces are thoroughly emulsified, with a needle or glass rod.
4. The emulsion is spread evenly over the slide so that a thin film of faeces is formed.
5. A Coverslip is put on the thin film and examined under the microscope with 10X objective lens for the presence of parasitic ova.

This rapid test is helpful when the infection is severe. Due to their weight and inability to float in many flotation solutions, some tapeworm, fluke, and whipworm eggs are particularly useful for this. Trophozoites and certain nematode larvae are found more frequently in wet mounts. It is possible to observe Trichomonas's motility.

B. Concentration methods

- These techniques remove the parasite items from the bulk of the specimen's material.
- There are two approaches. Flotation methods and the sedimentation method
- A combined of these two methods is also practiced.

1. Sedimentation method

Reliable for all type of parasitic eggs

- From different areas of the sample, a small amount of faeces (approximately 5 g) is thoroughly mixed with 10 to 15 ml of water (0.5 percent glycerine in water or 0.9 percent saline can be used for emulsifying the faeces instead of water).
- To eliminate larger particles, the emulsion is strained through a sieve.

- Centrifuge tubes containing the filtrate are filled just one inch below the brim and centrifuged at 1000 rpm for one to two minutes.
- A drop of the sediment is placed on a slide, covered with a cover slip, and viewed under a microscope after the supernatant is poured off (low and high power).

2. Flotation method

Because the eggs of trematodes, most cestodes, and a few nematodes cannot be floated up, this method is mostly useful for examining these infections.One can detect even a light infection by this method. In this method, a liquid heavier than the parasitic object is used to suspend the feces, causing the parasitic objects to rise to the surface and be skimmed off. The suspending medium must not only be heavier than the objects to be floated but also not produce any distortion in the objects to be examined. The commonly used suspending media are:

- Saturated salt solution (Sp. Gr. 1.18-1.19).
- A 33% solution of zinc sulphate (Sp. Gr. 1.18).
- A solution of saturated sugar (Sp. Gr. 1.25). Mix 355 ml of tap water with 454 g of granulated crystals. Add 7 ml of phenol crystals that have been liquefied and heat just until they dissolve. While too slow for simple floating, this solution is extremely suitable for centrifugation techniques.
- A saturated solution of sodium nitrate (to prepare a solution, dissolve 850 g of sodium nitrate in 1 litre of water and gently heat). The most eggs can be concentrated using this method.
- Glycerin.

1. Willi's technique

1. To create a convex surface, first fill a small floatation tube with a thick emulsion of faeces up to one-third of the way. Then, fill the remaining space in the tube with a saturated solution of sodium nitrate (or any other suspending medium) to the brim.
2. Hold it for an hour to give the eggs time to float.
3. Place a fresh cover slip on top of the fluid and withdraw just a drop of it for microscopic analysis. Alternatively, use a pipette or glass rod to scrape off the topmost layer of the fluid, place it on the slide, cover it with the cover slip, and study under the microscope.

2. Lane's method (centrifugal flotation)

- Put a small amount of faecal matter in a test tube.
- To emulsify the feces, add 10 times as much water.
- After passing the emulsion through a sieve, centrifuge it at 2000 rpm for 2 to 3 minutes.
- The sediment is once more suspended in water and centrifuged after the supernatant fluid is discarded. Up till the supernatant liquid is clear, centrifugation is repeated.
- Then suspend the sediment in a saturated sodium chloride solution, or in any other suspending medium, and centrifuge once more for 3 minutes at 2000 rpm.
- From the topmost layer, a few drops of fluid are taken, put on a slide, covered with a cover slip, and examined under a microscope.

The faeces may contain larvae (Lung worms) which may be found by concentration methods.

Negative results do not ensure the absence of parasites since the finding of eggs in faeces is dependent on many factors.

Reporting the results

No eggs are seen	Negative
Less than 1 egg per microscope field	Occasional
1 to 2 eggs/ field	1+
2 to 4 eggs/ field	2+
4 to 6 eggs/ field	3+
More than 6 eggs/ field	4+

Questions

1. Write name of quantitative tests of faecal examination?
2. Define flotation method of faecal examination?
3. Write name of methods of qualitative examination of faecal examination?

11

Laboratory Diagnosis of Protozoal Infection

Saurabh

A. Intestinal protozoa

Fresh faeces must be used as a sample. The sample must be examined immediately and without refrigeration.

Methods of examination

1. Direct smear examination

A thin smear of faeces mixed with either water or normal saline (recommended for Trophozoites since they stay intact and motile longer). Select blood-tinged mucus or tiny tissue bits if the faeces are dysenteric. One to two percent of an aqueous eosin solution can be used in place of saline or water, but the oocyst still resist the stain. The viability is examined using the eosin solution. It is possible to employ an iodine solution (which kills protozoa), which allows for the identification and differentiation of the protozoa. It is possible to diagnose amoebiasis, balantidiosis, coccidiosis, and histomoniasis.

2. Concentration method

This is employed when the cyst and other stages of intestinal protozoa are scanty.

i) **Sedimentation method**: Make a small amount of faeces from different portions. Make an emulsion by thoroughly mixing them with a suitable amount of water (or 5% glycerine in water or normal saline). Sieve it, then place the filtrate in a centrifuge tube and spin it for one to two minutes at 1000 rpm. Centrifugation must be repeated until the supernatant is clear. Remove the supernatant and use a microscope to examine a drop of the sediment on a slide.

ii) **Flotation method**: Make up an emulsion of a small quantity of faeces as mentioned above and sieve it. Take the filtrate and mix it with a flotation agent/suspending media like 33% zinc sulphate solution (of specific gravity 1.080) and spin it at 1500 to 3000 rpm for 2 to 3 minutes in order to bring the protozoa to the surface. Collect these with a wire loop or cover slip by lowering them on to the surface of the fluid and transferring the same on to a slide and examining them.

Faecal culture

Since each worm's larva has distinct diagnostic morphological characteristics, cultivating the faeces sample and examining the larvae is the only way to identify the specific causal parasite. There are two ways to perform faecal culture.

1. Watch glass or petridish technique
2. Barman's technique

1. Watch glass method

- Place a large lump of feces in a small petridish or watch glass. The faeces shouldn't be either too soft or too hard. If it's too hard, add additional water to make it soft. If the mixture is excessively soft or watery, add dry sterilised dung from the same species of animal or sterile normal animal charcoal in sufficient amounts to achieve the desired consistency.
- Put this dish or watch glass in a larger petridish filled with water (to the lip of the smaller petridish), cover the larger petridish with another dish or jar, and store it in a dark place at room temperature.
- Larvae that have hatched from ova and moved from the faeces sample will be abundant in the water in around 7 days. Numerous larvae would have progressed to the infectious stage, helping in specific diagnosis.

2. Baermann's Technique

When the larvae of particular parasites do not migrate, this method is employed. The apparatus is made up of a stand and a rubber tube with a funnel and clamps.

- Place wire gauze in a funnel on top of a tube.
- Add the faeces after covering the wire gauze with a linen cloth. Spread the faeces evenly.
- Fill a funnel with just enough water to cover the faeces. Leave it for two hours to stand.

- Eliminate the water from the funnel's bottom, where all of the larvae will be found.

Quantitative egg count technique

By counting the number of eggs present in one gramme of faeces, one can determine an animal's severity of infection or worm load. This is accomplished using two techniques.

1. Stoll's dilution egg count technique

Procedure

- Weigh 4 grammes of faeces and put them in a graduated test tube or small flask with a mark at the 60 ml level.
- If there is a lot of fat or mucus in the faeces, pour water up to the 60 ml threshold. N/10 sodium or potassium hydroxide is used instead of water (or 1 gram of faeces is taken and diluted with 15 ml of water or N/10 KOH or NaOH).
- Add small glass beads. With the lid securely fastened, shake the contents vigorously in a straight upward and downward motion for one minute, or until a homogeneous suspension is achieved. A hard faeces should be left in the liquid over night or till it dissociates when shaken. Avoid circular motion.
- Quickly discharge 0.15 ml of the suspension onto a clean slide using a calibrated capillary pipette (Stoll pipette).
- Cover the slide with a cover glass and mechanically move the slide to count all the edges of a certain type of helminthes under observation. The average of 2 such counts is taken.

This number is multiplied by 100 to obtain the number of eggs per gram of faeces (EPG).

2. Mac master method

The eggs are floated up in a counting chamber using this technique. The counting chamber consists of two glass slides that are separated from one another by three or four transversely placed strips of glass that are 1.5 mm thick. This creates two or three spaces of 1.5 mm depth between the two slides.

On the upper slide an area of 1 cm2 is ruled over each space.

- Weigh two grammes of faeces.
- Pour 30 ml of the saturated salt solution and mix well.

- Pour the contents of the filter into a glass jar and rinse the residue with an additional 30 ml of saturated salt solution.
- Completely agitate the sample, then take out a small amount (0.3 ml), filling both counting chambers.
- Nematode eggs predominantly float to the top. The trematode eggs collapse and are not float.
- Make several counts, and then arrive at the average of the results.

Depth of the chamber-1.5 mm

Dilution 2 g faeces in 60 ml (1:30 dilution)

Volume counted: 0.30 ml, i.e. 1/100th of 30 ml

Therefore the eggs counted multiplied by 100 gives eggs per gram

Similarly, a procedure may be followed for nasal discharge to get an EPG. If the amount is insufficient, they can be mixed with enough water or 5% formalin, centrifuged, and the sediment examined for specific ova.

Interpretation of EPG/ Ova per gram (OPG)

Nematodes

- Equines: 500- mild; 800-1000- moderate; 1500-2000-severe.
- Lambs: 2000-6000 severe
- Cattle: 300-600 severe

Trematodes

- Cattle: 100-200 of Fasciola- severe infection
- Sheep: 3000-6000 Fasciola- severe infection

Questions

1. Draw the eggs of worm parasite of cattle/ buffalo?
2. Draw the eggs of worm parasite of sheep and goat?
3. Draw the eggs of worm parasite of equines?

12

Examination of Skin Scraping

Saurabh

The essential database for all skin diseases consists skin scrapings. Skin scrapings fall into two main categories: superficial and deep. Superficial scrapings give information from the epidermis's surface without causing capillary bleeding.

Capillary haemorrhage is a sign that the sampling was deep enough to gather material from the hair follicle. Deep skin scrapings are used for this purpose. The main purpose of skin scrapings is to detect the presence or absence of mites. A skin-scraping spatula, which is a thin metal weighing spatula, is recommended for use while scraping the skin. These spatulas are safe and can be used again. Scrapings from active lesions at several places are to be submitted. Scraping from active lesions at several places is to be submitted. Generally, the periphery of the lesion contains more parasites than the centre. Skin scrapings are used to identify ectoparasites and fungal diseases.

Principle

If mange mites are present, both those that burrow in the skin (such as Sarcoptes) and those that live on the skin surface, they can be found by deeply scraping the skin surface with a scalpel blade held perpendicular to the surface (e.g. Psoroptes). The scraping needs to be deep enough to extract blood in order to enhance parasite recovery but not so deep that the animal dies. Before scraping, the scalpel blade is often dipped into a little amount of mineral oil. This helps in the material's adhesion to the blade, including the mites.

Requirements

- Diff-Quik stains
- Glass slides
- Coverslips
- Microscope - with low, medium, and high power settings (including oil immersion), and a high-quality
- Wood's lamp - needed for the skin scrapping experiments.

Methods of diagnostic tests for skin conditions

Coat brushing

This test can be used to check for ectoparasites, eggs, flea farces, and follicular anomalies, although it may go unnoticed in actual practise. The animal should be brushed either over brown paper or a black consulting table. It is necessary to gather the hair and epithelial debris and to separate the hair from the scale. The hairs are mounted in liquid paraffin with a cover slip for microscopic analysis and placed in a petri dish so they may be studied under the Wood's lamp. Additionally, liquid paraffin is used to affix the scale, and a cover slip is used. In cases of fleabite hypersensitivity, lice, nits, Cheyletiella, and fragmented flea faeces may be ignored macroscopically.

Hair plucks (trichoscopy)

An affordable and quick test for demodicosis is hair plucking, particularly on places like the foot where it is challenging to scrape the skin. From diseased areas identified by the dermatological examination, hairs are collected. Selective hair around the edges of lesions is pluck with tweezers, placed in liquid paraffin, and covered with a cover slip.

Skin scraping

Skin scraping takes a little longer than the earlier tests, but it is necessary when parasite involvement is suspected and less invasive tests come back negative. It is primarily used to identify surface and burrowing mites that transmit diseases like demodicosis and scabies, as well as other mites like Cheyletiella in some circumstances. The treatment for demodicosis is deep scraping. Should it be required, clip the hair. Apply liquid paraffin to the skin after gently pressing the skin in the area that will be scraped. The skin lubrication facilitates penetration and material collection.

Scrape in the direction of hair growth with a blunt blade. The initial scrapes may be superficial, followed by deeper ones (enough to cause capillary ooze). Material needs to be placed on a slide, mixed with liquid paraffin, and then covered before being examined at low power. Multiple superficial and deep scrapings in non-excoriated areas are needed to treat scabies. This is due to the fact that few mites may be present and many instances are linked to hypersensitivity to *Sarcoptes scabiei*. Only a small number of mites can be identified by scanning the slide at low power rather than high power. The mite is not killed by liquid paraffin, and little movements may be used to find its location.

Procedure of skin scrapping (if infection is mild)

- The Sample of skin scraping is boiled with 5 ml of sodium or potassium hydroxide in a test tube till a homogenous suspension is obtained. Allow it to cool.
- Pour this into a tube and centrifuge for 2 minutes at 1000 rpm.
- Pour off the supernatant
- Examine a drop of the sediment under the microscope for the presence of mites (or fungi).

Tape strips

Tape stripping is a highly effective and adaptable diagnostic procedure. It is rapid, affordable, and frequently provides useful diagnostic data. Since it can be utilised to identify superficial pyoderma, bacterial overgrowth, some autoimmune illnesses, and parasites, veterinary dermatologists frequently use this approach. The most popular method for identifying Malassezia dermatitis or overgrowth is tape stripping.A number of 10 cm strips of tape are applied to the skin's surface. Under low power, one sample is checked for parasites such Demodex, Sarcoptes, Cheyletiella, and lice. The tape is partially connected to the slide, stained with Diff-Quik, and then entirely attached for high-powered examination with oil immersion to identify bacteria or Malassezia. Ultra transparent tapes can be fixed without causing the tape to be damaged, and they typically produce better results.

Slide impressions and swab smears

Any purulent or exudative lesion should be examined using slide impressions of the lesion's surface. This method is useful for differentiating between bacterial infection and sterile lesions such as those seen in pemphigus foliaceus.

Low power is best for finding areas that can be examined under a microscope, whereas high power and oil immersion make it easier to identify bacteria and Malassezia. The glass slide is pressed against the moist lesion, fixed and stained with Diff-Quik. A swab can also be used to collect purulent material, such as material from pricked pustules, which is then gently rolled over the slide's surface.

Wood's lamp examination

A very helpful and affordable screening test for dermatophytosis caused by Microsporum canis is the Wood's lamp examination (other dermatophytes of veterinary significance do not fluoresce). The Wood's lamp must be of a high standard and come from a reputable veterinary supplier. It should emit UV light with a 253.7 nanometer wavelength. An inbuilt magnifying lens and two bars are features of high-quality Wood's lamps.

The examination must occur in a completely dark space. Give the lamp five minutes to warm up. For a few minutes, scan the animal because fluorescence can occasionally be delayed. Place the lamp over the gathered hairs from brushing. Only infected hairs glow, not surrounding skin or scale, and the apple greenish color is crucial for differentiating between true and false fluorescence. Positive fluorescing hairs can be pulled out, examined under a microscope, and confirmed through cultural examination.

Ectoparasites

Sarcoptes

The itch mite, also known as *Sarcoptes scabiei*, is an arthropod parasite that burrows into skin and causes scabies. The mite can be found everywhere in the world. Not only animals (like dogs and cats) but also humans are susceptible to infection. The body is globular or round in shape and smaller in size. The legs are shorter and do not project beyond the margins of the body.

Psoroptes: Several distinct animal species suffer from psoroptic mange due to the mite species Psoroptes spp. The mites do not significantly cause disease in wildlife, but they are a problem for domestic animals, particularly sheep. Psoroptes are bigger and elongated in shape. The legs are longer and project beyond the body margins. Only in males the coupulatory discs and tubercles at the posterior end are seen.

Demodex: *Demodex canis*, a parasitic mite that inhabits the hair follicles of dogs, is the cause of demodectic mange. This mite has eight legs and like a cigar under the microscope. The most typical type of mange in dogs is demodectic mange, sometimes known as "demodex" or "red mange."

Question

1. Draw the figure of Sarcoptes, Psoroptes Demodectic mite?

Appendix

Reagent/solution

1. RBC diluting fluid

a) **Gower's solution**

Sodium sulphate	2.5 gm
Glacial acetic acid	16.6 ml
Distill water	100.0 ml

b) Hayem's fluid

Sodium sulphate	2.5 gm
Sodium chloride	0.5 gm
Mercuric chloride	0.5 gm
Distill water	100.0 ml

2. WBC diluting fluid

a) For animals

Glacial acetic acid	3.0 ml
Distill water	97.0 ml

Add few drops of aqueous methylene blue to give colour to the solution

b) For birds:

Sodium citrate	3.8 gm
Formalin (neutral)	0.2 ml
Brilliant cresyl blue	0.5 gm
Distill water	100.0 ml

3. Benedicts reagent

Solution (a)

Sodium carbonate	100.0 ml
Distill water	800.0 ml
Dissolve by heating	
Sodium citrate	200.0 gm
Potassium thiocyanate	125.0 gm
Mix well and dissolve	

Solution (b)

Copper sulphate	18.0 gm
Distill water	100.0 ml
Dissolve by shaking	

Solution (c)

Potassium ferrocyanide	0.25 gm
Distill water	5 ml
Dissolve by shaking	

Mix the solution a, b and c at room temperature and make up the volume to 1000 ml with distilled water. Keep the solution in a dark coloured bottle.

4. Robert's reagent

Solution (a)

Magnesium sulfate saturated solution in distilled water

Solution (b)

Concentrated nitric acid

Working reagent

Solution (a)	5 parts
Solution (b)	1 parts

5. Sodium nitroprusside solutions

Sodium nitroprusside	10.0 gm
Distill water	20.0 ml
Dissolve by heating	

6. Biuret reagent

(Benidicts qualitative reagent)

Solution (a)

Cupric sulphate pentahydrate	17.3 gm
Distill water	100.0 ml

Solution (b)

Sodium citrate	173.0 gm
Sodium carbonate	100.0 gm
Distill water	800.0 ml

Dissolve by heating mix solution (a) and solution (b) and make it 1000 ml by distill water.

7. EDTA solution

Tetra sodium EDTA	5.0 gm
Distill water	100.0 ml

8. Zinc sulphate solution

Zinc sulphate	50.0 gm
Distill water	1000.0 ml

9. Iodine solution

Iodine crystals	2.0 gm
Potassium iodide	3.0 gm
Distill water	100.0 ml

10. Nessler's solution

Potassium iodide	30.0 gm
Iodine crystals	22.5 gm
Distill water	20.0 ml

Mix to dissolve. Add metallic mercury 30.0 gm. Dilute to 200 ml with distill water and mix it with 975 ml of 10% NaOH

11. Normal saline solution

Sodium chloride	0.835 gm
Distill water	100.0 ml

12. Lugol's iodine

Iodine crystal	1.0 gm
Potassium iodide	2.0 gm
Distill water	100.0 gm

13. Formal saline

35-40% formaldehyde	10.0 ml
Normal saline solution	100.0 ml

14. Buffered formalin

35-40% formaldehyde	10.0 ml
PBS (pH 7.2)	100.0 ml

15. Methylene blue stain

Methylene blue	0.03 gm
95% ethanol	30.0 ml
Distill water to	100.0 ml

16. Giemsa stain

Stock solution

Azure II- eosin	3.0 gm
Azure II	0.8 gm
Glycerol	250 ml
Acetone free methanol	250 ml
Working stain: stock solution	1 part
Distill water	9 part

17. Leishman's stain

Leishman's stain powder	0.15 gm
Methanol	100.0 ml

Mix in pestle and mortar. Filter before use

18. Lactophenol cotton blue stain

Phenol crystal	10 gm
Lactic acid syrup	10 ml
Glycerol	20 ml
Distill water to	10 ml
Cotton blue stain/ aniline blue	50 mg

Labs in India

S.No.	Veterinary Laboratory	Place
1.	Disease Investigation Unit	Goa
2.	Poultry Disease Investigation Lab	Gujrat
3.	District Disease Diagnostic Lab. Deptt of Animal	Haryana
4.	Chief Disease Investigation office Palode	Kerela
5.	Animal disease Research Laboratory, Khargone	Madhya Pradesh
6.	HSADL, Bhopal	Madhya Pradesh
7.	ADDL, Puducherry	Pondicherry
8.	Disease Diagnostic Lab	Rajasthan
9.	Disease Investigation Lab, Deorali	Sikkim
10.	Central Institute for Research on Goat	Uttar Pradesh
11.	Disease Investigation Lab Pashulok, Rishikesh	Uttrakhand
12.	Central lab, Tamilnadu	Tamil Nadu
13.	Poultry Disease Diagnostic Laboratory	Tamil Nadu
14.	ADDL, Adilabad	Andhra Pradesh
15.	ADDL, Bilaspur, H.P.	Himanchal Pradesh